Birthing Your Placenta
The Third Stage

Nadine Pilley Edwards
Sara Wickham

Association for Improvements in the Maternity Services

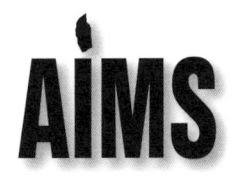

AIMS

©AIMS 2011
Third edition: fully revised
Published by AIMS
www.aims.org.uk

ISBN 978 1874413207

Printed in Great Britain by
QP Printing
www.qpprinting.co.uk

AIMS - Association for Improvements in Maternity Services

Acknowledgments

We would like to thank all those who have contributed to this booklet, especially those who, over many years, have carefully pieced together much of what we know about the birth of the placenta.

We would also like to thank the women who kindly sent us comments about their experiences of the time immediately after birth, and all members of the AIMS Committee for their input and unfailing support.

We extend huge thanks to Debbie Chippington Derrick, Jane Evans and Gill Gyte who made extensive comments on earlier drafts. Jane and Debbie spent many hours discussing and clarifying details of the third stage of labour. Also to Mavis Kirkham and Beverley Beech who made essential comments that we have incorporated into the booklet.

Our thanks too to Cath Pilley and Holly Lyne who proofread the final version and to Sam Farmer and Vicki Williams who proofread the references. We would also like to thank those who provided our artwork, Veronika Petrie, Sarah Montagu and Min White.

We are extremely grateful to Vicki Williams for layout and editorial support.

Cover illustration © Veronika Petrie.

Drawings and diagrams p14 and p16 © Sarah Montagu.

Placenta print p29 courtesy of Richard Grevers,
www.beautifulbellies.co.nz.

Contents

Introduction	1
Chapter One: Historical Background	7
Chapter Two: Development and Birth of the Baby and Placenta	11
Development of the Placenta	11
The Placenta	12
What Happens During and After Birth?	15
Leaving the Cord Unclamped and Uncut	19
Physiological Birth of the Placenta	23
Time and the Birth of the Placenta	28
Chapter Three: Actively Managed Third Stage of Labour	31
What Happens in Active Management of the Third Stage of Labour?	31
Uterotonic Drugs	34
Side Effects of Uterotonic Drugs	40
Cord Clamping and Cutting as Part of Active Management of the Third Stage of Labour	44
Controlled Cord Traction as Part of Active Management of the Third Stage of Labour	52
Chapter Four: Third Stage Research	55
The Bristol Third Stage Trial	58
Research Into Haemoglobin Levels	61
The Dublin and Brighton Trials	62
The Hinchingbrooke Trial	63
Subsequent Research	63
Systematic Reviews	64

AIMS - Association for Improvements in Maternity Services

Chapter Five: Wider Issues 67
    The Limitations of Existing Research 67
    Adaptations and Questions Arising from the Research 70
    Exploring Other Ways of Knowing 72
    The Impact of Setting and Practitioner Expertise 74
    A Note About Waterbirth 78
    Thinking Physiology 79
    Lotus Birth 81
    Women, Birth and Time 83
    How a Woman Feels During Placental Birth 85
    Placental Birth: Women and Decision Making 87
    A Final Word 90
    Post Script 91

Chapter Six: Resources and References 93
    Further Reading 93
    Useful websites 94
    Lotus Birth 95
    More Information 95
    References 96

A Note to International Readers

Although this booklet is written in the UK, we are aware that we have many international readers; women, midwives and others. We have sought to include enough detail to equip women in the UK with the knowledge that they need to make informed decisions. In order not to exclude readers from areas where practices, drugs, terminology and experiences may be different, we offer a few notes below as a quick guide to translation. The UK terms are explained throughout the following text

UK Terminology	Terminology used elsewhere
Uterotonic	Ecbolic
Syntocinon	Pitocin, Oxytocin
Ergometrine	Methergine, Ergonovine
Misoprostol	Cytotec
Carbetocin	Duratocin, Pabal

'Care for pregnant women differs fundamentally from most other medical endeavours. "Routine" care during pregnancy and birth interferes in the lives of healthy people, and in a process which has the potential to be an important life experience. It is difficult to imagine the extent to which our efforts might, for example, disturb the development of a confident, nurturing relationship between the mother and baby. The harmful effects we measure in randomised trials are limited to those we have predicted may occur. Sometimes after many years unexpected harmful effects surface only because they are relatively common, or striking in their presentation. Many unanticipated harmful effects probably never come to light.

'For these reasons, interventions in pregnancy and childbirth need to be subjected to special scrutiny. Our guiding principle is to advise no interference in the process of pregnancy and childbirth unless there is compelling evidence that the intervention has worthwhile benefits for the mother and/or her baby – only then is there a good chance that benefits will outweigh both known adverse effects and those which may not have been thought of.'

(Hofmeyr et al 2008, pxiii).

AIMS - Association for Improvements in Maternity Services

Introduction

The birth of the placenta is part of the awesome journey from woman to mother. For most women it follows closely on from the particularly precious moment when they meet their baby for the first time face to face.

> 'there are emotional, physiological, bacteriologic, hormonal and spiritual exchanges between the mother and the infant during this special time.' (Mercer and Erikson-Owens 2010, p82).

In many cultures, the placenta itself is an important and sometimes sacred organ, although it is also important to note that there are very differing perspectives on the significance, meaning and implications of this part of the journey of childbirth.

This booklet is for parents, midwives and others who would like to know more about the birth of the placenta, why there are ongoing discussions about the benefits and drawbacks of managing the third stage of labour or letting nature take its course, and what research and experience can tell us about the birth of the placenta.

The third stage of labour is usually defined as the period immediately following the baby's birth until the placenta and membranes have been born (Harris 2004). Physiologically, it involves the hormone oxytocin, which is produced naturally by a woman's body and is intimately linked with labour and birth. Over the past few decades, pharmacists have also developed synthetic forms of oxytocin which are commonly used within maternity care, although the synthetic form of oxytocin can interfere with a woman's ability to produce her own natural oxytocin (Foureur 2008). Oxytocin works by making the woman's womb (uterus) contract during labour, which brings

AIMS - Association for Improvements in Maternity Services

about the birth of her baby. As the baby is born, a further surge of oxytocin brings about the birth of the placenta. The woman continues to produce oxytocin after birth (especially when she is able to hold, cuddle and/or breastfeed her baby) and this oxytocin helps to keep her uterus contracted and blood loss controlled. In a natural third stage there is no interference with the process of placental birth and the placenta is birthed by the woman's own efforts. The amount of time that this takes varies from woman to woman.

The third stage is also described as the time when the *'activity and excitement accompanying the birth of the baby are replaced by the parents' quiet and wondrous contemplation of their offspring. The focus shifts from the mother's concentrated exertions to the miracle of the newborn. There is a sense of emotional and physical relief.'* (Sleep 1989, p209).

> *'it is hard to describe those first moments – such a mixture of joy and wonder and relief and curiosity about this new baby in your arms. And almost instantly it becomes hard to believe that they were ever in your tummy!'*
>
> Joanna Porter, Pregnancy and Parents Centre

As Jenny Sleep noted in 1989, this is a wondrous time for the parents as they meet their new baby, but she also suggested that

> *'...for the mother, this is the most dangerous stage of labour'* (Sleep 1989, p209).

The third stage of labour is seen by many caregivers as a time when they need to be especially attentive, and this is because of the potential for excessive bleeding during the birth of the placenta. This sentiment carries through subsequent editions of Myles Textbook for

Midwives (Sleep 1993, McDonald 1999, Fraser & Cooper 2003, Fraser & Cooper 2009) and it is because of this concern that, increasingly, women have been advised to have 'active management' for the birth of their placenta. Active management includes: the midwife giving the woman an injection of an oxytocic drug (uterotonic) as the baby is being born or immediately after birth; clamping and cutting the cord immediately after birth (within the first minute); and applying traction to the woman's end of the cord in order to birth the placenta soon after the baby's birth (controlled cord traction).

Yet, while there is certainly a need for watchfulness, as excessive bleeding after birth can be a major source of maternal morbidity and even mortality, this is not usual and occurs in only a small proportion of women. Thus active management of the third stage of labour is not of benefit to all women.

It is, of course, in the privileged context of a relatively affluent society where we have the means to treat unexpected bleeding that this booklet is written. In the UK, as in other high income countries, we are very fortunate that few women and babies die in childbirth – though of the very few women who do, excessive blood loss (often referred to as postpartum haemorrhage or PPH) after birth is still a cause (Confidential Enquiry into Maternal and Child Health 2007).

There is no way of eradicating all risk and the decision to enable the placenta to birth naturally is a reasonable one, particularly where the equipment and drugs to treat any excessive bleeding are available; and in the case of a home birth, where a hospital is accessible if necessary.

We do, however, have the disadvantage that birth in most parts of the affluent world has become increasingly medicalised, and some

AIMS - Association for Improvements in Maternity Services

women and babies suffer the side-effects of the overuse of medication and medical procedures, with both known and unknown effects. Like most interventions, active management of the third stage of labour carries risks and side effects (as discussed in Chapter Three on page 31). The third stage of labour is often accompanied by a significant level of fear. This fear is not always helpful, logical or designed to work in the best interests of mother and child. It does not always enable the birth attendant to focus on the woman and baby, or enable the woman to celebrate the birth of a new family member, which is so essential.

> 'I would say that nothing could have really prepared me for how wonderfully amazing it was to give birth to Finlay and finally hold him in my arms after nine months of excited anticipation. If I could re-live that day tomorrow, I would do it in a second because it was such an astounding time. I would like to be able to go back and savour each moment again. Although I had been told by other people, I hadn't truly appreciated the miracle of creating a person, which continues to amaze me, and the overwhelming love you feel for them.'
>
> Ros James, Pregnancy and Parents Centre 2010

> 'meeting our little girl was amazing; time seemed to stand still. She was a lot pinker and louder than I'd expected, and felt so fragile. I held her very close and wrapped her up in my arms – it was wonderful.'
>
> Mel Mere, Pregnancy and Parents Centre 2010

Fear can also have an impact on a woman's ability to produce her own oxytocin for labour and birth. In order for women's bodies to produce plenty of oxytocin they need to be in an environment where they feel safe and secure (Hastie 2011, Gurnsey and Davies 2010, Buckley 2009, Schmid 2005, Uvnas-Moberg 2003).

This booklet is intended to help women, midwives and others understand more about the third stage and the different approaches that may be taken. It is divided into several chapters. Chapter One discusses the historical background to the third stage of labour and further explains the differences between the approaches that different people take, Chapter Two describes the physiology of placental development and birth in more depth. Chapter Three goes into more detail about active management of the third stage of labour and Chapter Four looks at the research on this issue. Chapter Five examines other views about placental birth and looks at how women may decide to have a managed or physiological third stage, given the complexities of this topic. Chapter Six offers references and further resources.

Chapter One

Historical Background

It is impossible to know for sure how women birthed their placentas in ancient times and whether they had midwives who intervened (for instance with the use of herbs or physical manoeuvres) or who supported women in their own efforts, unless problems arose. We know that age-old beliefs existed in some cultures in relation to the meaning of the placenta, which sometimes led to traditions around the treatment and/or disposal of it after the birth. Some of these still exist today. We do not know whether, how and when ancient women separated themselves from their babies by biting or cutting the umbilical cord. Some people look to other mammals for an indication of this, only to note that there is some variation within the animal kingdom.

What we do know is that the vast majority of medical practices that exist in relation to the birth of the placenta today have become routine, and are based on the belief that women's bodies cannot be trusted, rather than on a good understanding of the physiology of the birth of the placenta. A good proportion of the medical treatments that are in use today are based on the needs of women who lived in societies and times when poverty and large family size would have made them more susceptible to excessive bleeding after birth.

We also know that the discovery of a fungus found on rotting rye (ergot) was one of the key developments in the history of the management of the third stage in labour. It was initially discovered that cows that ate this fungus were more likely to miscarry their calves, and it was learned that it works very quickly and is extremely effective at making the uterus contract. However, while midwives in the 17th and 18th centuries used this to treat bleeding after birth, they did so cautiously because it could cause spasms of the blood vessels which could lead to gangrene (Inch 1989, p147).

The third stage of labour started to be more systematically managed as medical men involved themselves more regularly in childbirth from the 18th and 19th centuries onwards. Ergot was first introduced into obstetric practice in 1807 but did not become popular until its reintroduction in 1932. By 1935 a new water-soluble ergot product had been isolated and was developed into a pharmaceutical product which became known as Ergometrine. Despite its side effects, like many other obstetric procedures, Ergometrine began to be used more frequently as a 'just in case' measure to prevent excessive bleeding, rather than for just the treatment of excessive bleeding. For more detailed information about its history see Baskett (2000), van Dongen and de Groot (1995), Inch (1989).

The 1950s saw the advent of a synthetic oxytocic drug called Syntocinon, which was hailed as a better alternative because it was thought that Ergometrine could cause retained placentas (Inch 1989, Begley 1990a). However, Syntocinon was not considered to be as effective as Ergometrine, and, in the 1960s, a drug which combined the two – Syntometrine – was developed. Both Syntocinon and Syntometrine are still in common use, and Ergometrine is also used in some circumstances. There is a range of other drugs to prevent or treat bleeding that have been developed and researched, and we discuss these in Chapter Four.

Along with the development of drugs, there has been a growth in the clamping and cutting of, and pulling on, the cord during the birth of the placenta. Some suggest that these interventions may have exacerbated problems during the third stage of labour (Mercer and Erikson-Owens 2010, Buckley 2009, Mercer, Skovgaard and Erikson-Owens 2008, Dunn 2004, Priya 1992, Dunn 1991, Inch 1989, Botha 1968).

It seems that, as the third stage of labour became increasingly managed, cutting the cord soon after the birth of the baby became normal practice. It has been suggested that this was so that the baby could be removed from the bed and the attendants could focus on the mother unhindered (Inch 1989). It is also thought that the practice of clamping the cord was developed because the quantity of blood escaping from the placental end of the cut cord could make a mess (Inch 1989). In a comprehensive review of third stage management, in her publication Birthrights, Sally Inch (1989) quotes Montgomery's view that these interventions might be due to the fact that:

> *'As the physician became more skillful with the use of haemostats, scissors and ligatures, the umbilical cord presented an inviting site for surgical procedures, and the present custom of immediate severance and immediate ligation of the cord followed. Ligation of the cord makes it possible to get babies and mothers out of the delivery room more rapidly, just as low forceps contribute to more rapid care. Whether they have added to the ultimate welfare of the newborn is a question.'* (Montgomery in Inch 1989, p166).

Montgomery's question continues to be pertinent and could still be applied to many aspects of maternity care. Despite the questionable value of routine active management of the third stage of labour, there has been a general assumption in practice that it is necessary and desirable for all birthing women, in order to facilitate the expulsion of their placenta and prevent excessive bleeding after birth. Recent research and discussion has tended to focus only on drugs and interventions during the birth of the placenta, for example: which oxytocic drug to use, when and how much of the drug to use, controlled cord traction (pulling on the cord), maternal effort (the woman pushing the placenta out herself) and fundal pressure (pressing on the woman's womb). Less attention has been paid to what measures, if any, might reduce the likelihood of too much bleeding occurring in the first place, such as good nutrition to support the woman's health and the growth of a healthy baby and placenta, appropriate birthing environments and skilled birth attendants.

This situation has, however, begun to change. While current guidelines in the UK (NICE 2007) support active management of the third stage of labour, they also recommend that: *'Women at low risk of postpartum haemorrhage who request physiological management of the third stage of labour should be supported in their choice.'* (NICE 2007, p183). The most recent Cochrane Review (Begley et al 2010) raises questions about the routine use of actively managed third stage for women who have had normal labours and births and who are not likely to bleed too much after birth. This may be an important development in the history of knowledge in this area.

Chapter 2

Development and Birth of the Baby and Placenta

Development of the Placenta

When a woman conceives, the fertilised egg travels down her fallopian tubes and implants in the wall of her uterus. Many complex processes take place and ultimately the egg forms into a growing baby with a placenta that is attached to the woman's uterine wall. The placenta enables the transfer of nutrients from the woman to her baby and the removal of waste products that the baby does not need. In nearly all cases, the egg embeds away from the woman's cervix (the neck of her womb) so that the placenta is well away from her cervix and her baby can be born vaginally. Women who have twenty week ultrasound scans are often told that their placenta is low. However, as the woman's uterus grows during pregnancy, most placentas will not be near the woman's cervix near the end of pregnancy. Placenta praevia, where the placenta is covering all or part of the woman's cervix is very rare and affects around 0.5 per cent of pregnancies.

The placenta is a beautifully evolved organ and the complex physical relationship between the woman, baby and placenta means that the mother's blood and the baby's blood do not directly mix during pregnancy or birth. Special structures and mechanisms develop in the woman's uterus and placenta to prevent the mixing of blood. These same special structures also have a role in the physiological birth of the placenta

The uterine muscle is also beautifully evolved and is unique in its elasticity and its ability to expand and contract during pregnancy, labour and birth. This elasticity is affected by the flow of oxytocin through a woman's body. It is the elastic nature of the woman's uterus that enables it to expand as the baby and placenta grow during pregnancy and to then reduce in size as the baby and placenta are born. Although it takes several weeks following birth for the woman's uterus to return to its non-pregnant size, in the vast majority of cases, a woman's uterine muscles will tighten immediately after the birth of her baby and placenta. This ensures that the part of the uterus to which her placenta was attached will be clamped down enough to prevent excessive bleeding in the first hours and days after birth.

THE PLACENTA

The placenta is roughly the size of a dinner plate. It usually weighs about a sixth to a fifth of the baby's weight and the umbilical cord is 50cms long on average. During the latter stages of pregnancy, the volume of the woman's blood flowing through the maternal placental site in any one minute is 500-800mls (Sleep 1993). About a third of the baby's blood volume is in the placenta (approximately 80-90 mls).

Following a physiological third stage, the surface of the placenta that was attached to the woman's uterus is smooth and shiny. Where active management of the third stage has been used, the placental surface appears dull and rough.

Many women are unaware that the placenta is their property and that they should be consulted in pregnancy about whether they would like to keep their placenta and/or what they would like to do with it. Occasionally women are distressed to learn later that they could have kept their placenta.

In the past, placentas were sold by hospitals to be used in cosmetics, but are now usually disposed of in hospitals by incineration. Sometimes caregivers may suggest that a woman's placenta is examined by a pathologist at the hospital because this can sometimes give useful information about her baby, for instance this may help determine whether twins are identical or non-identical. Midwives may want to take blood from the cord or placenta when women are rhesus negative and there is a need to find out what the baby's blood group is. In some areas, blood is taken or drained from the placenta and cord and may be used to check the baby's oxygen levels, or may be used in research or in the treatment of some diseases. Women can withhold consent to procedures, including immediate clamping of the baby's cord.

There is a growing interest both in the placenta as an extraordinary organ which nourishes the baby during pregnancy, and in the rituals surrounding it in other cultures

(Priya 1992). Some parents are redeveloping their own rituals in the UK, for example, planting a tree, bush or plant over the placenta. Occasionally, a woman may cook and eat her placenta, or have it raw, in an attempt to avoid postnatal depression, possibly due to the hormones contained in it, or just because of its nourishing qualities. It is also becoming popular in some areas to gently dry the placenta and make capsules of placental extract which is also considered nourishing. Placentas may also sometimes be used to make a homeopathic remedy.

We know of many women who have wanted to keep their placenta and some women decide they would like to keep their placenta attached to the baby until it falls off naturally; a practice known as lotus birth (see page 81).

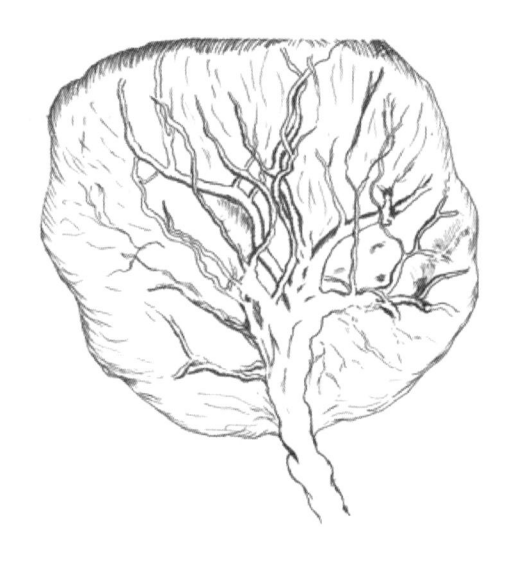

What Happens During and After Birth?

The placenta provides the baby with oxygen and other substances while it is in its mother's uterus and during the first few minutes, or more, after birth. At the birth of the baby there is a redistribution of blood from the placenta to the baby. It is for this reason, among others, that there is a growing practice of not clamping or cutting the cord until it is clear that the transfer of blood between the baby and its placenta has ceased, and this is discussed below.

Once the baby has been born, the placenta will continue to function until it separates from the uterine wall. This process happens very quickly in some women and much more slowly in others – just as in other stages of labour. Disturbing the woman at any time during her labour can slow or stop her labour, and many people have noticed that if a woman is disturbed around the time of birth, the separation and birth of the placenta can be much slower and may result in complications. This may well be because adrenaline, the hormone that is produced under such circumstances, interferes with the ability of the woman's body to produce the oxytocin that facilitates the birth of the placenta as well as the baby.

During the birth of the placenta itself, strong uterine contractions cause the woman's uterine wall to contract making her placenta peel away (Sleep 1993). It is generally thought that the placenta folds in on itself and the contracting upper part (or segment) of the uterus causes it to fall into the lower segment of the woman's uterus. Simultaneously the muscle fibres in the upper segment of her uterus (sometimes referred to as 'living ligatures') are able to clamp the exposed uterine blood vessels due to the pressure of her rapidly shrinking uterus. Meanwhile the woman's cervix remains open and if she is upright, the placenta meets little resistance and falls into her

AIMS - Association for Improvements in Maternity Services

vagina and is expelled, usually aided by gravity, by the woman's pushing efforts (Kierse 1998) and by the release of oxytocin in the mother (especially likely if her baby nuzzles or feeds at her breast).

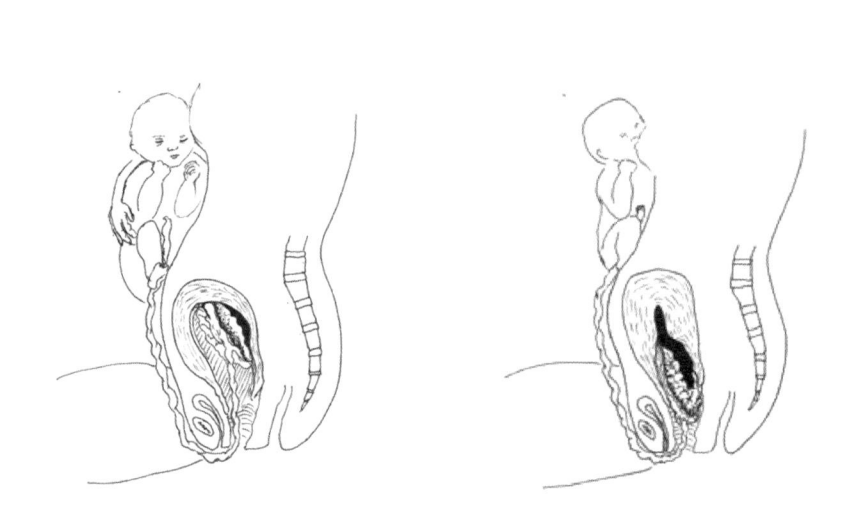

Separation of the placenta

A natural or physiological birth of the placenta is sometimes also referred to as 'passive' or 'expectant' management of the third stage. Throughout this book, however, we have talked more about the birth of the placenta rather than the third stage, especially when we are talking about the birth of the placenta under natural circumstances. This is because (a) we feel it is important to acknowledge that it is women who give birth to both their baby and their placenta (whereas 'management' is something that is done to women by others), and (b) the artificial division of labour into stages that has emerged as part of the medical view of childbirth is not necessarily representative of how women themselves experience this journey. Furthermore, a number of people, including Michel Odent (1998b) have pointed out that a physiological process does not need to be 'managed'.

French obstetrician Michel Odent (1998b) believes that when labour and birth have been normal, without induction or acceleration of labour with synthetic hormones, without pharmaceutical pain relief (pain relieving drugs), without instrumental delivery (forceps or ventouse), and when the woman can remain undisturbed and adopt whatever position she pleases, there is usually no need to induce or accelerate the birth of the placenta either. While there is no bleeding there is no need for haste. More recently, the Royal College of Midwives (RCM 2008) has suggested that physiological third stage *'can be seen as a logical ending to a normal labour.'* (see page 23).

A number of changes occur as a baby is born and in the first minutes of its life which help it to adapt from life inside its mother's womb to life outside the womb. In the past it has been widely assumed that the baby only needs air in order for its lungs to expand and for it to begin to breathe on its own. However, researchers have been aware for several decades that babies adapt more easily and are healthier if their cords are not clamped immediately at birth (Mercer et al 2000). This suggests that the transition that they make is more complex than first thought and that their dependence on their placentas does not end abruptly at birth. More recently we have begun to understand how complex the physiology of the transition from the mother's womb is. In particular we now understand much more about the importance of the baby's blood during this transitional process.

While in its mother's uterus, the baby's lungs produce amniotic fluid and are not filling with air, thus do not need much circulating blood. At any given time, a relatively small amount of the baby's blood circulates in its lungs (about 8-10%). The placenta, on the other hand, requires a constant flow of blood and around 40% of the baby's blood is circulating in the placenta throughout pregnancy (Mercer 2001).

At birth, the function of the baby's lungs changes from producing fluid to opening and being able to fill with air so that the baby can breathe on its own. In order for this to happen most easily, the baby needs much more blood to flow to its lungs (about 45% of the total). This flow of blood to the baby's lungs helps the air sacs (alveoli) in the lungs to expand so that air can flow in and fill them (Mercer and Erikson-Owens 2010, Mercer et al 2008, Mercer 2001).

Total Blood Volume

Age	Example Weight (kg)	Approximate Total Blood Volume (ml/kg)	Estimated Total Blood Volume (ml)
Premature infant	1.5	89-105	134-158
Term newborn	3.4	78-86	265-292

Approximate total blood volume information compiled from Nathan and Oski's Hematology of Infancy and Childhood, 5th ed. Nathan DG and Orkin SH, eds. (1998) Philadelphia, PA: WB Saunders.

Reprinted from www.pediatriccareonline.org/pco/ub/view/Pediatric-Drug-Lookup/153949/0/Total_Blood_Volume

Leaving the Cord Unclamped and Uncut

'Another thing very injurious to the child is the tying and cutting of the navel string too soon: which should always be left till the child has not only repeatedly breathed but till all pulsation in the cord ceases. As otherwise the child is much weaker than it ought to be, a portion of blood being left in the placenta which ought to have been in the child.' (Darwin 1801).

If the baby's umbilical cord (from now on referred to as the cord) remains unclamped and intact for a while after birth, blood continues to flow through it from the placenta in the minutes after birth and it continues to pulsate. If the cord is clamped at birth, this blood cannot flow through it and the blood is therefore unavailable for the process of lung expansion. Blood then has to be 'borrowed' from the rest of the baby's circulation in order for its lungs to become fully functioning, even though the baby's other organs also need blood to start to function fully (Mercer and Erikson-Owens 2010, Mercer et al 2008).

If the cord is clamped very soon after birth, this also means that the oxygen that would have continued to support the baby through the pulsating cord immediately after birth is unavailable. When the baby's cord is left unclamped and intact, it will usually only stop pulsating when the baby has made a successful transition and is well oxygenated (Mercer 2001).

> 'Max was very slow to breathe, but his cord continued to pulsate strongly. I instinctively rubbed him whilst my midwife cared for him in my arms. He slowly started to breathe and after a few minutes he became more alert, his breaths became less shallow and more regular, and his grey colour changed to pink. I often wonder if my bright intelligent boy would be with us today if his lifeline had been cut.'
>
> AIMS anon

We do not know exactly how long the cord should be left unclamped and intact, but to clamp it before it has stopped pulsating and before the placenta has been born is clearly a disruption to the physiological process. Because this practice is so wide-spread, there is a belief by some practitioners that, despite the fact that immediate clamping of the cord is an intervention, it should remain the status quo until leaving the cord unclamped has been shown to be safe. Obstetrician David Hutchon (2010) suggests that this is part of the reason why obstetricians and midwives have been resistant to changing their practice on cord clamping. Many experienced midwives feel that because we do not know enough, it is best to leave the cord as long as it practical. The woman's contractions continue after the birth, and while the placenta is being born, and this helps the flow of blood to the baby (Mercer and Erikson-Owens 2010, Mercer 2001). If the baby is above the placenta, blood tends to flow a bit more slowly, and if the baby is below the placenta it tends to flow a bit more quickly into the baby (Mercer and Erikson-Owens 2010, Mercer et al 2008, Mercer 2001).

A common misconception has been that the baby is getting 'extra' blood or 'blood overload' (Mercer and Erikson-Owens 2010) if its cord is left unclamped and intact. Over the years, many practitioners have believed (and many still believe) that this 'extra' blood could cause problems such as polycythaemia and hyperbilirubinaemia (both of which are associated with too many red blood cells in the blood). Three key things that we have learned in recent years are that:

1. This blood should not be thought of as 'extra' or 'unnecessary' as the blood in the placenta is the baby's blood. It plays a hugely important role in the baby's transition to life outside the womb.

2. During and after birth, a number of complex physiological processes take place which we are only just beginning to understand. But these depend on our not interfering with the cord immediately after birth, in order to allow the baby's body to maximise its transition to life outside the womb. There is no clear evidence that letting the baby receive its full quota of blood results in any harm. The Cochrane Review (Begley et al 2010) found mixed results regarding the likelihood of jaundice in babies born to women who had physiological third stages.

Jaundice in newborns is still under debate and requires further research. There is growing evidence that not interfering with this part of the process is better for the baby (Mercer and Erikson-Owens 2010, Mercer et al 2008, Mercer 2001).

3. Polycythaemia (increased red blood cells) and hyperbilirubinaemia (an excess of bilirubin; a pigment created by the break down of red blood cells) could possibly arise if the baby is held too low immediately after birth and an unnatural amount of blood might transfer to the baby.

Almost a third of babies are born with the cord looped around their neck one or more times. Mostly it is not very tight and will not prevent the baby being born, yet many practitioners want to clamp and cut the cord when this occurs. It is strongly recommended by Judith Mercer and colleagues (2010, 2001) that practitioners should wherever possible leave the cord unclamped and intact, loosen the cord and loop it over the baby's head, or use the 'somersault manoeuvre' to release the baby's cord from around its neck. This is particularly beneficial if the baby's cord is wound tightly around its neck, as the baby may have experienced some reduction in oxygen and may be even more in need of its full quota of blood. Even if the cord looks empty of blood initially, it will usually refill as the placental circulation will continue.

If the baby needs any resuscitation at birth, Judith Mercer and colleagues suggest that wherever possible this should be done next to the mother with the cord unclamped. In the rare situations where for some reason, it is necessary to clamp and cut the baby's cord immediately, they suggest quickly 'milking' the baby's cord (Mercer and Erikson-Owens 2010, Mercer et al 2008). This means holding the umbilical cord and using thumb and fingers to sweep down the cord from the placental end towards the baby, up to four times. This moves blood from the placenta quickly into the baby. There are interesting anecdotal experiences of this quoted in a chapter by Judith Mercer and Debra Erikson-Owens in Soo Downe's edited book, Normal Childbirth: Evidence and Debate (2008). This technique may also be used by experienced practitioners where the baby is 'slow to start'. However, there needs to be further research on this technique to be clearer about any benefits and harms.

While a healthy baby will almost always manage to make the transition to life outside its mother's womb without obvious harm, even if its cord is immediately clamped, there are numerous short and long term benefits to leaving the baby's umbilical cord unclamped and uncut. For a baby who is already compromised, leaving the cord unclamped can provide the baby with crucial advantages, while clamping the cord can leave a baby seriously further compromised. Cord clamping is discussed further on page 44.

Physiological Birth of the Placenta

There appear to be important advantages to physiological placental birth unless there are specific reasons for active management of the third stage of labour. These include:

- Avoiding all the disadvantages (known and potential) to women and babies associated with active management of the third stage (see Chapter Four).

- Eliminating the sense of urgency and anxiety about birthing the placenta within the time frame associated with active management.

- Once the baby is born, a calm and quiet atmosphere can be maintained. This enables everyone present to appreciate and experience the wonder of birth and to welcome the new baby. Undisturbed, the mother can focus on her baby in her arms and enjoy skin-to-skin and eye contact. She will thus be in the best possible hormonal balance to stimulate the necessary release of natural oxytocin to expel the placenta (Buckley 2009, Schmid 2005, Odent 1998b).

- The woman's sense of confidence in her own body may be enhanced.

If a woman plans to birth her placenta naturally it is important that:

- The woman and midwife should have fully discussed different options for the birth of the placenta, including the advantages and disadvantages of these options and when they may be appropriate, along with the physiology of normal labour.

- The woman is able to adopt the positions she finds most comfortable. It is our experience that it is preferable for women not to be advised to adopt a particular position during any part of labour and birth unless their caregiver feels that there is a specific reason to do this, for example, to avert or deal with a potential problem. This maximises women's ability to trust that their bodies will almost always instinctively know how to facilitate labour and birth better than an external observer.

- Labour or birth has not been induced or augmented using oxytocic drugs, or interfered with in any other way. Because the administration of synthetic oxytocin will inhibit a woman's ability to produce her own natural oxytocin, it is not advisable to aim for a natural placental birth following the administration of any uterotonic drug.

- The woman and midwife recognise the benefits of putting the baby to the breast and thus stimulating the woman's body to release oxytocin. It is important to note that this is an advantage rather than an absolute necessity. Breastfeeding is not a prerequisite for a natural third stage: if the baby 'nuzzles' near its mother's breast or if she cuddles her baby, this will have a similar effect on the woman's oxytocin levels (Foureur 2008). Also, even if this is impossible for some reason, this does not preclude physiological birth of the placenta.

- The midwife recognises the signs of placental separation and descent, and is sensitive to the possible causes if placental separation seems to be delayed. If the baby is not present for some reason, nipple stimulation could be tried by the woman, her partner, or other person that she trusts to touch her in this way.

- Just as in earlier phases of labour, emotional factors may delay the process and the woman may need patience and quietness to let her placenta go and make the final transition to motherhood (Edmunds 1998). It is important that she does not feel observed by those around her (Odent 1998b).

- The woman should be kept warm and comfortable, as blood loss is associated with higher levels of catecholamines (stress hormones). The woman may produce these if she is too cool (see Odent 1998b for further comment).

For more detailed information about the physiology of the separation and expulsion of the placenta, and the different components of active and physiological approaches to the third stage of labour, a number of midwives with a particular interest in this aspect of labour and birth have written informative chapters in midwifery textbooks and books for women. See, for example, Mercer et al (2010), Buckley (2009), Mercer and Erikson-Owens (2008), Sweet (1997), Sleep (1993), Levy (1990) and Inch (1989).

There is a growing body of work, mainly written by midwives, which is exploring the finer details of facilitating physiological placental birth. This work includes discussion of tips, 'tricks' and remedies that can be used if, for instance, the birth of the placenta needs to be expedited for some reason. Some sources of this work include the 'Tricks of the Trade' books published by Midwifery Today (www.midwiferytoday.com) and journals such as Midwifery Matters (www.midwifery.org.uk) and Birthspirit Midwifery Journal (www.birthspirit.co.nz) which tend to focus on low-tech midwifery and the skills that go along with this.

Whether or not complications arise depends on a variety of factors. The woman's general health and energy levels and whether or not she is genuinely anaemic are important. The skill of those attending the birth in facilitating the natural birth of the placenta, detecting developing problems, preventing or treating bleeding, protecting the woman from infection, detecting retained placenta and preventing or treating shock are equally important.

Based on his own work and observation, Michel Odent suggested that certain principles may positively facilitate the birth of the placenta, and at the same time enhance crucial bonding processes between mother and baby. The facilitation of the birth of the placenta and bonding processes occur because of the release of certain hormones – most notably, oxytocin, commonly known as the 'hormone of love'. They can only occur however, if the mother and baby are in a warm room, and there is undisturbed contact between them. He believes that quietness and privacy are essential (Odent 2002, 1998a,1998b). Experienced midwives are continuing to develop and articulate a midwifery approach to the birth of the placenta which takes into account: the health of the mother and baby, how birth has unfolded, the environment for birth and the psychological and emotional factors that might impact on the mother birthing her placenta (Fahy 2009).

Another issue is that, for a variety of reasons – including the fact that many hospitals encourage women to have a medically managed third stage – some midwives are neither comfortable with, nor experienced in helping women to birth their placenta naturally. In one study (Featherstone 1999), using one particular definition of physiological placental birth, only 33% of midwives appeared to understand this process. Eleven years later, Diane Farrar and her colleagues (2010) showed that only 2% of UK obstetricians and 9% of UK midwives always or usually facilitated physiological placental birth. According to Izumi Featherstone, when describing their practice, 10% of midwives unknowingly described potentially unsafe practices. These practices included omitting to give an oxytocic drug but then applying all other components of active management during a physiological placental birth. Such practices are known to increase the likelihood of excessive bleeding. Women often report that midwives attending births in the community (which includes independent midwives and NHS community midwives) tend to be more likely and able to facilitate physiological placental birth.

AIMS - Association for Improvements in Maternity Services

Time and the Birth of the Placenta

There can be considerable variation in the length of time between the birth of the baby and the birth of the placenta where this occurs naturally. While up to one and a half hours is considered within the normal range (Cronk & Flint 1989), many of the midwives who regularly attend physiological placental births report waiting for much longer with no adverse effects. One account describes a breech baby arriving unexpectedly at home, wearing its placenta like a 'floppy hat' (Wesson 2006, p124), while other anecdotal accounts tell of the placenta being born many hours after the baby's birth – in one case, 48 hours.

Occasionally, the placenta is embedded in the woman's uterus in such a way that it will not come away naturally, and partly because of this there has been debate over the years about the maximum safe length of time for the third stage. Most often, the policies in place in maternity care systems recommend waiting only half an hour to an hour for the placenta to be born, because it is believed that the likelihood of bleeding increases after this time. One midwife researcher said that she knows of no evidence to intervene after an hour if time is not a constraint, and that the decision to intervene after one hour is often a purely pragmatic decision in busy maternity units (Jane Rogers 1999, personal communication). As far as we are aware, this has not changed.

There is some suggestion that it is when women have received active management of the third stage of labour that they are more likely to bleed if there is a delay in the placenta being born (Begley et al 2010).

It is also important to remember that caregivers cannot give drugs or perform manoeuvres without the consent of the woman, and some women choose to wait longer, as long as they are not experiencing bleeding or other problems.

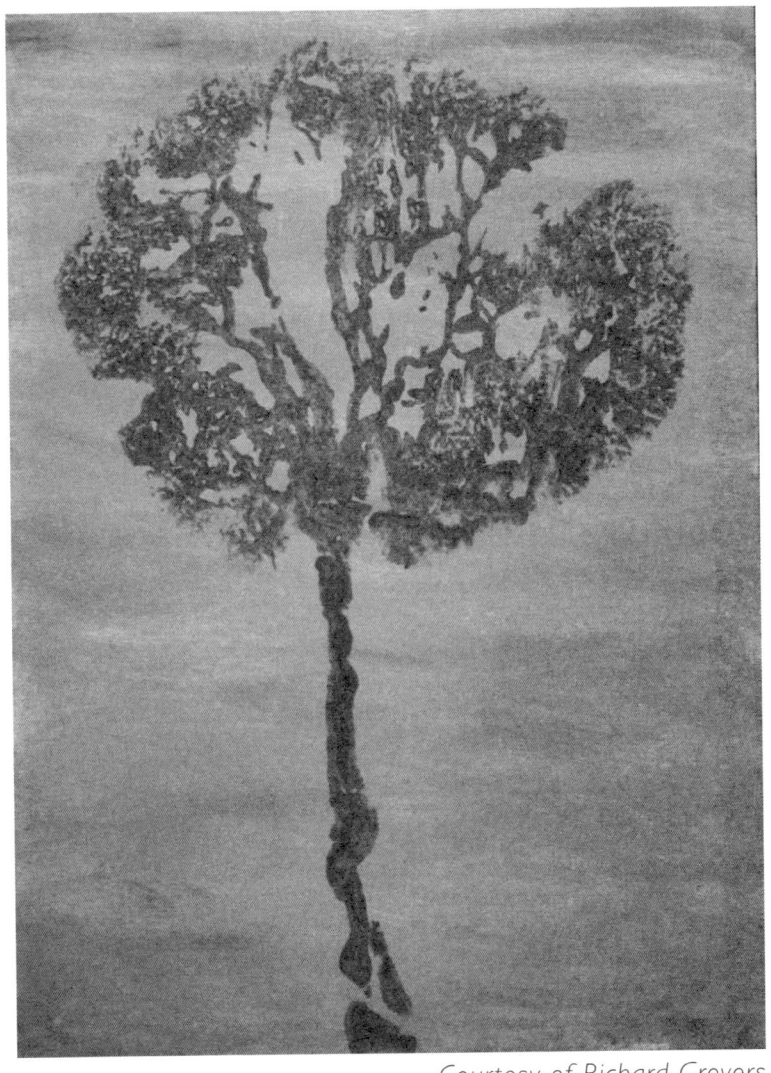

Courtesy of Richard Grevers

Chapter Three

Actively Managed Third Stage of Labour

Active management of the third stage of labour is routinely recommended in nearly all hospitals in the UK in line with NICE guidance (NICE 2007). It is considered by most medical and many midwifery professionals to be beneficial because some research has suggested that it reduces blood loss and shortens the third stage of labour. The most recent Cochrane Review (Begley et al 2010) suggests that there are benefits and harms associated with active management of the third stage of labour. It also suggests that we need to consider previous research on this in more detail, and acknowledge its uncertainties, along with its demonstrated harms as well as benefits. Our experience at AIMS to date, however, has been that changing strongly held beliefs and practices happens only very slowly, especially when these are part of a more medicalised view of birth. Research on the third stage of labour is discussed further in Chapter Four.

What Happens in Active Management of the Third Stage of Labour?

When the third stage of labour is actively managed, in most countries, a uterotonic drug is given by intramuscular injection (these drugs are discussed below), the cord is usually clamped and cut immediately after the baby's birth and then the placenta is delivered by controlled cord traction.

Controlled cord traction (often referred to as CCT) is a specific manoeuvre to deliver the placenta. It is carried out relatively quickly once an oxytocic has been given. The midwife will usually place her hand on the mother's abdomen so that she can feel when the woman has a contraction. One study suggested that it is advantageous to wait until the cord has lengthened and a fresh trickle of blood has been seen, which indicates that the placenta has separated from the uterine wall (Levy & Moore 1985). However, once an oxytocic has been given, the placenta must be delivered within a few minutes to avoid retained placenta. The midwife then uses sustained traction (pulling) on the cord, whilst guarding the woman's uterus by applying pressure with her hand to ensure that the woman's uterus does not become inverted during the procedure. An inverted uterus is one that turns inside out and comes into, or even outside, the woman's vagina. The woman is usually lying down or in a semi-reclining position as it is then easier for her attendants to apply the different components of active management. This is not always the most comfortable position for the woman to adopt at this stage. The midwife might have also placed a container under the woman to catch and assess blood loss as she is delivering the woman's placenta.

When uterotonic drugs are given it is usually assumed that the placenta needs to be birthed within a relatively short length of time. In cases where there is a delay, the woman is often advised that it needs to be removed manually in order to avoid a retained placenta. If this occurs, the woman will be offered an epidural, spinal or a general anaesthetic and it is unlikely to be carried out for at least an hour or so after birth. However, experienced midwives have suggested that in cases where there is a delay, even after an actively managed third stage, a woman's cervix will sometimes eventually relax and open of its own accord to allow the birth of the placenta (Cronk & Flint 1989). Although it is not common practice in Britain to take a 'wait and see' approach following a managed third stage, we know of a number of cases where women who were scheduled to have their placenta removed under anaesthetic have managed to push their placentas out once the effect of the uterotonic drugs have worn off. Having a manual removal and the associated anaesthetic can entail disadvantages to the woman's health and her ability to bond with, feed and generally care for her baby immediately after birth.

Although managed third stage is used internationally, a consistent approach does not exist. In some places it is considered bad practice to give uterotonic drugs before the birth of the placenta (for example, in the USA and in France) while in others it is considered bad practice to undertake controlled cord traction without having given an uterotonic (for example, in the UK). A study that compared the administration of intravenous oxytocin before and after the birth of the placenta showed no significant differences between the two approaches (Jackson et al 2001). However, this study considered intravenous oxytocin and in most cases oxytocin is injected into a muscle rather than intravenously and there is thus a need for further research and discussion around this issue.

Typically the third stage is said to last around 5-15 minutes when it is actively managed (Sleep 1993). The 'speed' of a managed third stage is often used as a 'selling point' when options are discussed with women. However, some women who birth their placentas naturally do so very quickly too. There are some important questions about whether speed and urgency really are the key goals here and how this impacts not only on the baby's successful adaptation to independent life, but also how it impacts on the new family's need to spend time together peacefully, immediately after the birth of their baby.

Management of the third stage of labour, like many other interventions in labour, was introduced without research which considered the full impact of the intervention on the mother and baby. Over the last decades, a growing number of researchers, midwives and parents have questioned many interventions including whether or not active management of the third stage of labour should be routine for all women.

Some have suggested that the woman's individual health and circumstances should be taken into account and that the effects of uterotonic drugs and other components of active management on the woman and baby should be given more consideration. The Cochrane Review (Begley et al 2010) confirms that these are important questions to raise. It has looked carefully at the known and potential harms caused by active management of the third stage of labour, as well as its benefits for women who are more likely to bleed too much or who do experience heavy bleeding at birth.

Uterotonic Drugs

A uterotonic drug is one that causes the uterus to contract, and this class of drugs includes the oxytocic drugs which we discussed above and which are synthetic forms of the naturally occurring hormone oxytocin. All uterotonic drugs are powerful substances which stimulate uterine contractions. Undoubtedly, oxytocics and other uterotonic drugs have saved the lives of many women and will continue to do so. They are effective in dealing with bleeding in most cases.

There are two different ways of using uterotonic drugs during the third stage of labour. The first is when they are used as a treatment for excessive bleeding. The second way of using them is as prophylaxis – or as a preventative measure – as in the case of routine active management of the third stage of labour

Much of the research that we discuss in this section assumes that these drugs will be used as a part of routine active management; that is as prophylaxis rather than treatment. Currently, in the UK most women who are given oxytocic drugs receive them as part of routine active management, rather than as a treatment for excessive bleeding during physiological placental birth.

As we discussed in Chapter One, management of the third stage has tended to involve the use of uterotonic drugs, including Syntocinon and Syntometrine, but some newer drugs (including Carbetocin, another oxytocic and Misoprostol, a prostaglandin-like drug) are being used and researched, and these are discussed below.

- Syntocinon is a synthetic oxytocic which acts within about four minutes when given intramuscularly.

- Syntometrine is a combination of Syntocinon and Ergometrine. A 1ml vial of Sytometrine is made up of 5mg of Syntocinon and 0.5mg of Ergometrine. Ergometrine is a uterotonic which acts within 6-7 minutes when given intramuscularly. Both Syntocinon and Ergometrine work faster when given intravenously, but Ergometrine is not usually used on its own or given intravenously in the UK because it can cause potentially harmful side effects (Liabsuetrakul 2007).

One of the reasons that the combined preparation (Syntometrine) became popular is that it combined the quick but shorter-lived effect of Syntocinon with the slower but stronger and more sustained action of Ergometrine. It is not, however, appropriate for women with pre-existing high blood pressure because Ergometrine can cause a further raise in blood pressure. In such cases, practitioners have tended to use Syntocinon on its own.

There is growing evidence to support the trend of using Syntocinon on its own rather than Syntometrine within the context of a managed third stage and this is now recommended by NICE (2007). However, anecdotal evidence suggests that some midwives, because they are used to giving Syntometrine, are applying controlled cord traction too early and may be contributing to increased blood loss when using intramuscular Syntocinon. Greater patience and more time appears to be required when intramuscular Syntocinon is used. A number of research studies and analyses (Orji et al 2008, McDonald et al 2004, McDonald 1999) have compared these preparations and shown that, if a woman chooses an actively managed third stage, there is no evidence of a difference in blood loss over 1000mls between Syntocinon and Syntometrine, but Syntocinon has fewer side effects. As a result of this research, it is becoming far more common for practitioners to use Syntocinon during managed third stage.

A much wider debate has been occurring in relation to other drugs that can and might be used during managed third stage and/or to treat bleeding. Below we discuss newer preparations that are being researched.

Misoprostol

Over the past few years, researchers have been examining the use of a drug called Misoprostol (a prostaglandin-like drug) in preventing and managing bleeding after birth, in the hope that this might be a safer, more stable and cheaper alternative to oxytocics. Unlike Syntocinon and Syntometrine, Misoprostol does not need to be kept in a cool, dark place, which is another potential advantage, particularly in hot countries and especially where refrigeration is not always available.

The findings of research have, however, been very mixed, and more research is needed before any firm conclusions can be drawn (Gülmezoglu et al 2007). Misoprostol can either be given rectally or orally but researchers have studied a wide range of dosages and compared these with different routes and doses of oxytocic drugs, so the results, as the following summary shows, are difficult to compare.

The studies involving Misoprostol have produced wide-ranging and contradictory results:

Studies on rectal misoprostol

- Diab et al (1999) found that 200µg (micrograms) and 400µg of rectal Misoprostol were both better than an intramuscular oxytocic.

- Wangwe et al (2009) and Gertensfield and Wing (2001) found 400µg rectal Misoprostol to be as effective as intramuscular and intravenous oxytocin respectively.

- Caliskan et al (2002) found that 600µg of rectal Misoprostol was less effective than oxytocin.

Studies on oral misoprostol

- Ng et al (2001) and Cook et al (1999) showed that 600μg and 400μg were less effective than an oxytocic.

- Many studies, however, have shown that Misoprostol is as effective (Parsons et al 2006, Zachariah et al 2006, Garg et al 2005, Vimala et al 2004, Caliskan et al 2003, Walley et al 2000) if not more effective (Singh et al 2009) than an oxytocic.

- Dosages in these studies have varied (mostly between 400μg and 800μg).

An overall view of the research would tend to suggest that, if Misoprostol is going to be useful, it is probably more effective to continue to research giving this orally rather than rectally.

A recent review (Gülmezoglu et al 2007), incorporating a larger number of studies, concluded that:

'Misoprostol orally or sublingually at a dose of 600mcg [micrograms] shows promising results when compared to placebo in reducing blood loss after delivery. The margin of benefit may be affected by whether other components of management of the third stage of labour are used or not. As side-effects are dose-related, research should be directed towards establishing the lowest effective dose for routine use, and the optimal route of administration.

'Neither intramuscular prostaglandins nor Misoprostol are preferable to conventional injectable uterotonics as part of the management of the third stage of labour especially for low-risk women.' (Gülmezoglu et al 2007, p1).

Misoprostol does have side effects (see page 40) and – whether or not they found it effective in their setting/study – a number of the researchers who have looked at this area believe that more research is needed (Vimala et al 2004, Hofmeyr et al 2001). There seems to be a consensus that Misoprostol is only justifiable as the drug of choice during a managed third stage where alternatives may not be viable, affordable or otherwise available (Gülmezoglu et al 2007, Zachariah et al 2006, Ng et al 2001, Walley et al 2000). We have included a significant amount of detail on this issue, because we understand that, despite this consensus, women are sometimes being given Misoprostol as a part of active management of the third stage of labour in settings where oxytocics are easily available. A recent Cochrane Review (Gülmezoglu 2007) suggests that Misoprostol is effective enough to be useful where injectable oxytocics are not available but that it has side effects – the most common are shivering and high temperature. Misoprostol is sometimes also used for induction of labour, but a recent Cochrane Review (Hofmeyr et al 2010) suggests caution as it results in more women suffering harmful, strong, very long contractions one after the other (hyperstimulation of the uterus). The authors' concern is clear from a highlighted sentence in their conclusion: *'The authors request information on cases of uterine rupture known to readers.'* Misoprostol is not approved in the UK for induction, or for use during the third stage of labour.

Carbetocin

One other drug that is currently being tested for use in managed third stage of labour is Carbetocin. Early research in this area is suggesting that intramuscular Carbetocin may be as effective as intramuscular Syntometrine and it appears that it is less likely to induce high blood pressure and has fewer side effects in the women who receive it (Su et al 2009, Leung et al 2006). So far, however, only a few relatively small studies have been undertaken and more research is needed. It may be interesting to note that the results of early studies into a number of other drugs, including Misoprostol, have suggested that they were more promising than they actually turned out to be.

All of the uterotonic drugs discussed in this section may also be used as a treatment when women bleed more than is considered ideal, and more research is needed in this area too. However, many practitioners consider the non-evidence based use of drugs such as Misoprostol, Carbotocin and Carboprost, which are still undergoing evaluation, to be more justified when there is excessive bleeding, especially if a woman continues to bleed following standard treatment with oxytocic drugs.

Side Effects of Uterotonic Drugs

The disadvantages and side effects associated with the use of the drugs to manage the third stage of labour in healthy women experiencing normal labours have been, and continue to be, discussed.

Some of the disadvantages and side effects associated with the use of uterotonic drugs include:

- Common side effects of Syntometrine include nausea, vomiting, headaches, tingling of the limbs, dizziness, ringing in the ears, palpitations, pains in the back and legs and raised blood pressure (Inch 1989). Raised blood pressure, along with after pains necessitating analgesics, and women returning to hospital with bleeding after being discharged were specifically mentioned in the Cochrane Review (Begley et al 2010) as some of the disadvantages of Syntometrine and active management.

- The woman and her midwife are in a race against the clock to birth the placenta before the cervix closes, as a result of the drug used, possibly leading to a retained placenta.

- Uterotonic drugs do not prevent all cases of excessive bleeding from the placental site, and there are other reasons for bleeding during the third stage. For instance, a woman may bleed from an episiotomy (see Inch 1989 for further comment) and bleeding may also occur if a woman has torn during her birth.

- Very rare complications of Syntometrine include cardiac arrest (heart failure), intracerebral haemorrhage (bleeding in the brain), myocardial infarction (heart attack), postpartum eclampsia (high blood pressure and possible fits after birth), pulmonary oedema (fluid on the lungs) and, in some rare cases, these have led to the woman's death (see Inch 1989).

- Though extremely rare now, intrauterine asphyxia (lack of oxygen) may occur when an undiagnosed twin is present because the Syntometrine is given with the anterior shoulder of the first baby – the death rate in this situation for the second twin is 35%, and few escape unscathed (Inch 1989). The use of scans has reduced this unusual incidence, but cannot eradicate the possibility completely, and some women do not wish to have scans because we are still unsure about the impact of ultrasound on unborn babies (Beech and Robinson 1994).

- Though very rare, injections can be mixed up. We know of one case where neonatal convulsions were caused in a baby given an oxytocic drug instead of Vitamin K, and another where a baby died when a mother was given Syntometrine instead of pethidine when she was in labour.

- Syntometrine affects smooth muscle (these are involuntary muscles such as the uterus, heart and stomach) and is usually given in the UK as the baby is being born, while the cord is still intact, and therefore reaches the baby. It is thought by some, that this might be implicated in causing colic in babies.

- In 1990, a study by Begley (1990) showed that women who did not receive Ergometrine during the third stage of labour breastfed their babies for a longer period of time. This was thought to be specific to this study in Ireland where Ergometrine had been given intravenously. Ergometrine on its own was not, and is not, routinely used in the UK for the third stage of labour. Oxytocin was assumed not to have any impact on breastfeeding. However, recent research suggested that, *'Oxytocin and ergometrine in the third stage of labour ... were associated with a significant reduction in breastfeeding rates ... analyses suggested that reduced breastfeeding rates were associated with intramuscular oxytocin (5 units) in combination with ergometrine (500µg) ... Ergometrine alone was associated with the greatest reduction.'* (Jordan 2009 quoted in Buckley 2011, p38).

- Almost all of the studies involving Misoprostol found that its use was associated with side effects, most notably shivering, raised blood pressure and raised temperature (Hofmeyr 2001). Women who were given Misoprostol have also been found to experience nausea, vomiting and diarrhoea, persisting for several hours after giving birth (Lumbiganon et al 2002).

- The side effects of Carbetocin require further evaluation but, because this is an oxytocic, they are likely to be similar to the side effects of Syntocinon. Carboprost has also been found to cause vomiting and diarrhoea.

- The use of any uterotonic drug nearly always goes along with further interventions which carry inherent risks of their own, such as early cutting of the cord and controlled cord traction because we do not know which, if any, of these interventions reduce bleeding, or if a uterotonic drug on its own might be just as effective as the whole package of active management (Begley et al 2010).

As Jean Robinson noted in the foreword to the original version of this booklet:

'When randomised trials report on outcome from any extra intervention, they do not mention the additional risks each one brings. With every drug comes a risk that it will be given to the wrong person in the wrong dose or at the wrong time. And drugs given by injection are riskier than those given orally, since their diverse effects are likely to be more severe, and they can be injected into the wrong place as well as the wrong person. For additional procedures, each new intake of staff has to practise and learn on someone – like the mother whose cord was broken when the medical student was told to practise controlled cord traction.

Those of us who often dip into medical literature, soon realise that adverse effects of intervention often surface only when a different treatment becomes available for comparison. Proponents or producers of the new drug or treatment will then happily write about the disadvantages of the old, in order to convert colleagues to the new. This is also true of different oxytocic drugs used to reduce haemorrhage risk in the third stage.' (Robinson 1999, p8).

Cord Clamping and Cutting as Part of Active Management of the Third Stage of Labour

'Early cord clamping had no specific rationale, and it probably entered the protocol by default because it was already part of standard practice. When this package was shown to reduce postpartum haemorrhage in the 1980s early cord clamping became enshrined in the modern management of labour.' (Weeks 2007, p312).

During active management of the third stage of labour, the cord between the woman's placenta and her baby is usually clamped in two places and then cut between the two clamps immediately after the baby's birth. The midwife then applies controlled cord traction (as described above) to make sure the placenta is born before the woman's cervix closes. Whenever the cord is cut at the baby's end, it should be cut at least 3-4 cms away from the baby's body to avoid pinching the skin or clamping a portion of the baby's gut which may in rare circumstances protrude into the cord. A swab or gloved hand should be held over the cord as it is cut to prevent mess from the small amount of blood that will remain between the clamp and the place where the cord will be cut.

There is an increasing trend in some areas, during active management, to leave the cord unclamped and intact for longer. The World Health Organisation recommends that women be offered active management of the third stage of labour, but also recommends *'delayed cord clamping to allow baby's blood that is in the placenta to return to the baby's circulation through the cord to reduce the likelihood of anaemia.'* (Begley et al 2010, p2).

In days gone by, it would probably have been unnatural for a mother to cut the umbilical cord quickly. She would have been unlikely to have anything with which to cut it. In some animals, the cord remains untouched after birth and is then severed some time later.

Obstetrician MC Botha tells us that he observed 26,000 births over a ten year period among the Bantu women in Africa (Botha 1968). According to Botha, these women gave birth in a squatting position and the cord was left completely untouched until after the birth of the placenta and membranes. Although he said that he saw many complications during this time he seldom witnessed a retained placenta and a blood transfusion was never given for a postpartum haemorrhage. British professor in perinatal medicine, Peter Dunn, during his extensive work in the field of third stage management made similar observations (Dunn 1991). A Dutch doctor argued that nature cannot usually be improved upon and attempts to do so without cause can be detrimental to mother and child (Kloosterman 1975). This call to do no harm has since been repeated by many of those concerned about the impact of interventions on the physiological process of pregnancy and birth (see, for example, Wickham and Robinson (2010) and the quote by Justus Hofmeyr and his colleagues at the start of this booklet).

AIMS - Association for Improvements in Maternity Services

Researchers reviewing the literature suggested that, even as late as 2000, there was no sound research on the timing of cord clamping to guide parents and practitioners, but that early clamping and cutting of the cord was still widespread practice, especially when babies are compromised (Mercer et al 2000). Paradoxically, the babies who are most likely to have their cord clamped and cut quickly are the very babies who would benefit most from having their cords left intact and unclamped. We now know, as explained above, that early clamping and cutting of the cord has a number of potentially serious, undesirable side-effects for term and preterm babies which have been well researched and documented.

Many of these serious disadvantages occur because of the reduced volume of blood and red blood cells that the baby receives around the time of birth, as well as the sudden removal of the baby's oxygen supply, when the cord is clamped quickly. When a baby receives its full quota of blood, it is able to maintain its haematocrit levels (ratio of red blood cells to total volume of blood) better (Yao & Lind 1974). In the past, commentators knew that this quota of blood was important (see Inch, 1983) but it is only recently that we have come to understand the implications of early cord clamping more fully. Judith Mercer (2001) has suggested that clamping the cord early can lead to a reduction in blood volume of up to 30% and a reduction of red blood cells of up to 60%. The Cochrane Review (Begley et al 2010) suggests that about 20% of their blood volume is lost to babies whose cords are clamped early. In both early and more recent studies there is inconsistency in the actual amount of blood volume that babies receive if the cord is left pulsating. While this ranges from 50-165mls, the average is around 80mls (Begley et al 2010). A baby's total blood volume is 80-90 mls per kilogram in weight. Very recent research (Farrar et al 2011) involving twenty-six babies showed that babies who received placental blood were from 87g to 116g (depending on how this was measured) heavier than babies who did not and that they gained from 83ml to 110ml of blood. This meant that babies whose cords were not clamped gained about 32ml of blood volume per kilogram of birth weight and that this 'equates' to 24%-40% of *'total potential blood volume'* (p70). The authors also noted that: *'Placental transfusion was usually complete by 2 minutes, but sometimes continued for up to 5 minutes.'* (p70). The loss of blood through early cord clamping can result in:

- Lower iron stores and anaemia in babies. This is particularly serious in low income nations but can impact on babies wherever they are born. Judith Mercer and Debra Erikson-Owens (2010) point out that, *'iron deficiency is the most common nutrient deficiency in the world and is a problem for babies and small children as they need iron to grow.'* (p87). They go on to suggest that this can impact on myelination (an important part of the development of the nervous system) and thus brain development during the first year of childhood and that the effects of this can continue into adulthood (Mercer and Erikson-Owens 2010, Mercer 2001). It appears that reduced blood volume and red blood cells at birth can therefore impact on both short and long term health and development.

- Increased levels of intraventricular haemorrhage (bleeding into the brain) and infection, which is not only potentially serious in the short term, but can also impact on later development (Mercer and Erikson-Owens 2010).

- Fewer stem cells going to the baby at birth. Stem cells have miraculous healing qualities, and when the baby's cord is clamped and cut at birth, the baby receives almost a billion fewer of these cells (Mercer and Erikson-Owens 2010).

- Less 'protected' time (Mercer and Erikson-Owens 2010). When the cord is clamped at birth, the baby has to adjust to life outside the womb without the protection and support of blood and thus oxygen that would have continued to flow through its cord.

While severing the baby's lifeline quickly and suddenly can have detrimental effects on some term babies, the effects can be even more detrimental in babies who are premature (particularly if born by caesarean section) or who are slow to breathe at birth (Mercer and Erikson-Owens 2010, Mercer et al 2008, Mercer 2001, Mercer et al 2000, Dunn 1991, Dunn 1989). In addition to all the impacts of reduced blood volume, red blood cells and stem cells already noted, these babies are more likely to need oxygen, ventilation and blood transfusions and are more likely to suffer from respiratory distress (breathing difficulties), intraventricular haemorrhage (bleeding in the brain) and sepsis (widespread serious infection).

In addition early clamping of the umbilical cord can result in:

- The possibility of the placenta being bulkier when fetal blood is prevented from passing to the baby (Dunn et al 1966) – at the time of this research it was suggested that this might prolong placental separation due to fetal blood remaining in the placenta which may delay retraction (shrinking) of the woman's uterus.

- Increasing blood loss in the woman (Botha 1968) – though there is mixed evidence on this issue, it has been suggested that clamping the maternal end of the cord may interfere with placental separation and predispose a woman to a blood loss (Levy 1990, Wood and Rogers 1997).

- Increasing the possibility of feto-maternal transfusion (mixing of the baby and mother's blood) because of a larger volume of blood remaining in the placenta. As the uterus attempts to contract to expel the placenta, the pressure exerted can cause placental vessels to rupture, allowing fetal cells into the maternal system. This may be critical if the mother is Rhesus negative and her baby is positive (Wickham 2001, Prendiville and Elbourne 1989, Lapido 1972). Rogers et al (1998) considered this in their research but did not confirm an association.

- It is suggested by Inch (1989) that when blood in the placenta is not given time to drain because of clamping the cord quickly and leaving it clamped at the maternal end, there is the possibility that extra blood clots will form in the woman's uterus, providing an ideal environment for infection. She and Jenny Sleep (1993) suggest that stagnant blood may also be left in the stump of the baby's cord which provides another place for infection to develop – though a subclinical (mild) degree of infection of the cord stump is normal and is thought to facilitate its separation.

Until relatively recently it has often been assumed that most healthy babies tolerated early clamping and cutting of the umbilical cord without harm, We now have more detailed knowledge about the baby's transition from inside to outside its mother's womb, that questions this assumption. Michel Odent (1998b) and others suggest there may well be other short and long term impacts that have not been thought about yet, for both women and babies. Further research is still needed. However, we now know of a number of wider benefits associated with delaying clamping of the cord, as follow:

- The woman and her baby can remain undisturbed to allow the natural physiological processes which assist placental separation and birth to occur. Remaining undisturbed can enhance the relationship which begins to develop between the mother and her baby and between the woman's partner and their baby, if he or she is present. Siblings may also be present and will also be meeting their sister or brother for the first time. The first hour or so after birth is a particularly awesome, miraculous, important, delicate and intense time of transition for mother, baby and family. If undisturbed, both mother and baby will continue to produce hormones that help them to form a strong, loving bond. This helps the woman to feel protective of her baby, and according to physiologist and midwife Verena Schmid (2005), contributes to ongoing attachment patterns between mother and baby, between family and baby and in the baby's ongoing relationships, as it moves through childhood into adulthood.

- The mother and baby are more likely to have skin to skin contact and the baby is likely to nuzzle and begin to suckle at its mother's breast. This improves the baby's oxygen levels and lowers its heart rate (Mercer and Erikson-Owens 2010). It also increases the flow of the hormone oxytocin, which helps the separation of the woman's placenta and is the main hormone of love (a term first used by Niles Newton (see Foureur 2008)) and bonding (Schmid 2005, Odent 1999). It might also prolong early breastfeeding from 10-12 days (Mercer 2001).

- The placenta continues to function, carrying blood rich in oxygen to the baby after birth, helping with both its breathing and circulation (Mercer and Erikson-Owens 2010). This is advantageous, particularly if the baby is premature or asphyxiated (deprived of oxygen) because this leads to a reduction in respiratory distress, the need for oxygen and ventilation and blood transfusions (Mercer 2001, p402), as well as a reduction in sepsis (widespread infection) and intraventricular haemorrhage (bleeding in to the brain). (Begley et al 2010, Mercer and Erikson-Owens 2010).

- Furthermore, when the baby's cord was left unclamped and uncut, babies had higher iron levels at two months of age, and some also had higher iron stores at six months of age (Mercer and Erikson-Owens 2010). Research suggests that delaying clamping and cutting of the cord *'can provide adequate iron stores for the first 6-8 months of age.'* (Mercer and Erikson-Owens 2010, p87). This is especially important where poverty means that ill health and lack of food and good nutrition are common.

- It has been suggested that the stump of the baby's cord may separate more rapidly postnatally (see Sleep 1993), especially when it is left intact for some time, as with a lotus birth (see page 81).

Controlled Cord Traction as Part of Active Management of the Third Stage of Labour

Controlled cord traction is believed to contribute to a shorter third stage. It is applied as part of active management of the third stage of labour after an oxytocic drug has caused a strong uterine contraction following the baby's birth, and once the placenta appears to have separated from the woman's uterine wall. The recent Cochrane Review (Begely et al 2010) on third stage management suggests that we do not know if controlled cord traction, as part of active management contributes to reducing blood loss at birth. It may even increase the likelihood of secondary bleeding (bleeding at a later stage) after birth.

Problems associated with the use of controlled cord traction include:

- The risk of pulling out a placenta that has not yet completely separated, which could lead to further bleeding immediately after birth, and may create the need for the placenta to be manually removed and/or the risk of infection.

- The possibility that it might leave small pieces of the woman's placenta or membranes behind, and this could be the cause of secondary bleeding (bleeding at a later stage). This is more common in women who have had active management of the third stage of labour, and often occurs after the woman has been discharged from hospital (Begley et al 2010).

- The cord occasionally being snapped or pulled off. If an oxytocic has been given and the midwife is unable to reach the woman's end of the cord and there is a delay in the third stage, the woman's placenta may need to be manually removed (though it may still be birthed by the woman if attendants are patient).

- The risk of causing the woman's uterus to invert partially or fully, even when the midwife guards her uterus. This is rare and can also happen when oxytocics have not been used for the birth of the placenta, but is more common when controlled cord traction is used (Inch 1989, Cumming and Taylor 1978).

- Causing the woman pain if the placenta is not completely separated.

All the above can happen when the placenta is completely healthy and normal. However, occasionally the placenta may have grown with an extra lobe or the cord can be attached right on the edge of the placenta. In both of these situations, controlled cord traction may be more likely to cause a problem than if the placenta is allowed to birth naturally. We are aware of situations where midwives have been very glad that a woman chose to have a physiological placental birth because the cord and/or placenta was fragile and may not have remained intact if controlled cord traction had been used.

However the third stage is managed, any pressing, pushing or other handling of the uterus ('fundus fiddling' or 'fundal fiddling') can be painful for the woman and occasionally results in additional bleeding. Although this should be avoided in the absence of a problem, it is important to note that, if a woman is bleeding, firmly massaging her uterus will encourage it to contract and thus reduce bleeding.

Chapter 4

Third Stage Research

Within the medical literature, there is no discussion of 'placental birth'; all of the research and discussion focuses on the 'third stage' of labour. This emphasis reflects the importance that is placed on discrete and measurable stages of labour and birth and observing and managing birth from the perspective of an outsider. It fails to appreciate the centrality of personal experiences or the active involvement of the women in the process. This chapter explores the research that has been carried out on the management of the third stage of labour and we have reverted to the terminology used in the original studies. This is because much of the research defines labour into stages, as though they are unrelated to each other, rather than an integral and inter-connected element of the woman's birthing journey. The research also focuses on the 'management' of women, and it would be inappropriate to continue to talk about placental birth in a chapter which discusses work that has often been carried out in environments where women are frequently unable to 'own' their experiences.

The research in this area is limited; it focuses on short-term physical outcomes rather than taking a more holistic approach, and hence considers a limited range of physical outcomes. One of the biggest problems with many of the research studies is that they consider the amount of blood that a woman loses during and immediately after the birth of her placenta to be the key factor in determining which kind of approach is best. If a woman loses more than 500ml of blood, she is commonly considered to have had a postpartum haemorrhage.

There is a lack of consensus about how much blood constitutes a postpartum haemorrhage, but even if there was a consensus, research consistently shows that it is incredibly difficult to accurately estimate or measure blood loss (e.g. Schorn 2010) not least because blood tends to mix with other fluids (such as amniotic fluid) and soak into sheets, pads and other fabrics.

However, haematologist Gill Gyte (1992) suggested that it would be more useful to consider haematological and physical implications of third stage management rather than blood loss alone. She also suggested that healthy women appear to cope well with blood losses of up to 1000mls, and that we know very little about the consequences of either very small or heavy blood loss during third stage. This point was also made by the Cochrane review (Begley et al 2010).

One of us (Sara) regularly speaks to large groups of midwives about placental birth, with the following experience:

> 'I often ask the midwives present to put up their hands if they have seen a woman lose more than 500mls of blood and be fine. Almost everybody raises their hands. Then I ask them if they have seen a woman lose more than 1000mls and be fine; again, almost all the hands go up, and finally I ask if they have seen a woman lose less than 500mls of blood and be compromised. Quite a few midwives raise their hands at this point too. We have to understand that the measurement of blood loss alone is not helpful. We also need to look at how the woman copes with that blood loss on physical and other levels, and base decisions about transfer (in the case of a home or other out-of-hospital birth) and treatment on the basis of how the woman is rather than on an arbitrary and often inaccurate measurement of how much she bleeds.'

It goes without saying that if blood loss results in women feeling exhausted in the weeks after birth, this is detrimental to both mother and child. As the above quote shows, this may occur even in the absence of a large bleed, and if women are not feeling well then they should ensure that they get appropriate attention whether or not their blood loss was considered 'normal'.

There has been a growing tendency towards redefining normal blood loss. Historically, a post-partum haemorrhage was defined as a blood loss over 500mls, yet it has been suggested that this amount of blood loss does not have a detrimental effect on a woman who is well nourished (Bloomfield and Gordon 1990). It is also worth noting that this is the standard amount of blood that is removed during blood donation (Burnley et al 2006) and that because of blood dilution that occurs during pregnancy, this equates to around 600-750ml of blood after birth (Begley et al 2010, p21). In addition, good blood dilution (haemodilution) during pregnancy lessens the effect of bleeding.

More recently, postpartum haemorrhage has been defined as where a woman loses more than 1000mls of blood (Begley et al 2010), yet even 1000mls is not thought to be necessarily excessive in a well-nourished healthy population, and does not need treatment if the woman is well (World Health Organisation 1996). During pregnancy, a woman's blood volume will increase by 1000-1500mls, and a number of people have asked whether it might actually be detrimental to try and reduce women's blood loss around the time of birth. It seems logical that, once the baby and placenta have been born, the woman will not need this excess of blood.

It is interesting, but perhaps not helpful, that Western medicine has focused almost entirely on seeing blood loss as pathological, whereas, around the time of birth, the loss of a reasonable, but not excessive amount of blood is normal and healthy. Again, we would not want to define 'reasonable' in solely quantitative terms, but in relation to the woman's well-being.

One final point is that many of the trials that we discuss in the following pages have used the term 'expectant management' rather than 'physiological third stage'. We have also used this term as it reflects the fact that, in these settings, even a placental birth that occurs without the use of drugs or manoeuvres is often still 'managed'. The women in all of the studies discussed below gave birth in hospital. This kind of setting will not necessarily provide the kind of environment conducive to the flow of birth hormones, which raises a number of questions about the accuracy of the findings in relation to the outcomes of physiological third stage. One of the studies that is most needed is one which looks at the experiences of women who give birth at home or in home-like settings with midwives who are skilled at facilitating the birth of women's placentas in a way that is supportive of this as a normal and natural journey (see page 74).

The Bristol Third Stage Trial

Because the results of research into third stage management were contradictory and confusing, in 1986 researchers planned and executed a large trial in Bristol. This was designed to show whether or not active management of the third stage should be routinely recommended to all women (Prendiville et al 1988). The results were published in the British Medical Journal and were considered to be authoritative and definitive by many doctors and midwives.

The authors concluded that active management should continue to be routinely recommended, as blood loss in the women receiving physiological management was significantly higher.

Criticisms of the Bristol trial appeared in both professional and lay journals following the publication of the results. These included that:

- The hospital already had a policy of recommending routine active management of the third stage and, prior to the trial, only six weeks had been allocated for the midwives to become familiar and confident in using a physiological approach. At the start of the trial only 13% of the midwives felt very confident in expectant management, and this went up to only 22% after the trial (Begley et al 2010). There is ongoing debate about whether or not this affects outcomes (Featherstone 1999, Kierse 1998, Stockdale 1997). However, in a trial by Cecily Begley and colleagues (1990) the postpartum haemorrhage rate in the expectant management group dropped over the course of the trial from 21% in the pilot study to 12% over the first four months to 7% in the last six months as the midwives became more experienced at facilitating women to give birth to their placentas naturally (Begley et al 2010). This may have dropped even further had the midwives continued to gain experience.

- Women who were already at increased risk of bleeding were included in the Bristol trial. (This includes women who had not experienced normal first and second stages of labour, women at known risk of postpartum haemorrhage, women who were given opiate drugs and women who had episiotomies.) All of these women should have been excluded from the research because this does not give a true result for expectant management in women who had a low risk of excessive bleeding after birth. The argument used was that the researchers did not know for certain if these reasons were justifiable reasons for recommending active management. They should however have divided the women in the study into sub groups (stratified) before the randomisation so that we could have looked at the outcomes for these groups of women separately.

- A large number of women (53%) who should have had physiological third stages had neither physiological nor active management. They received a mixed approach including components of active management such as clamping the cord and early cord cutting. In some cases, a physiological approach seemed only to mean avoiding the use of Syntometrine (Gyte 1991, Gyte 1990, Inch 1990, Stevenson, 1989). It is thought that omitting the uterotonic whilst continuing with the other components can increase risk of excessive bleeding.

It is interesting to note that both women and midwives involved in the trial preferred active management of the third stage (Harding et al 1989). This is not surprising considering this had been the midwives' usual practice for years, and was a practice with which they were very comfortable. Also, because the Bristol trial was a randomised controlled trial (RCT), women who had already stated a preference about the third stage of labour were automatically excluded from the trial, and this would have included women who were motivated to have a normal birth.

More recent research suggested that women were satisfied with whichever form of third stage management they received (Rogers et al 1998). This appears to support the notion that women believe that 'what is must be best' (van Teijlingen et al 2003, Porter & MacIntyre 1984) and that many women assume that any care offered must have been well thought out (Santalaahti et al 1998).

There was much debate about the methodology and findings of Bristol trial. Some of the trials we discuss in the following pages did make clear attempts to respond to some of the problems identified in this trial. Thus one of the achievements of the Bristol trial was that it raised many questions and stimulated thinking in this area.

Research into Haemoglobin Levels

Around the same time as the Bristol trial, midwife Barbara Watson carried out a small, retrospective research project involving 100 women at a hospital in England. Half of the women experienced a physiological third stage and half had active management. This research found that haemoglobin levels after three days were similar among all the women in the trial and concluded that a physiological third stage is appropriate for some women (Watson 1990). At the time of the research this hospital already had a physiological third stage rate of 17%, therefore the midwives were already relatively competent and confident with this approach.

This study used haemoglobin levels rather than blood loss as a term of reference. As we suggested before, it may be much more helpful to consider women's well-being (partly though haemoglobin levels) than blood loss per se (although the impact of, for example, shortness of breath, tiredness, dizziness, fainting, ability to care for the baby would be best), and estimates of blood loss are frequently inaccurate, with a tendency towards underestimation when blood loss is high, and overestimation when blood loss is low (Razvi et al 1996).

The Dublin and Brighton Trials

These trials included women who were considered to be well and at low risk of bleeding.

The Dublin trial was carried out by midwife Cecily Begley in Ireland (1990a). Intravenous Ergometrine was used as the oxytocic for woman having managed third stage, which is not normally used in the UK. The results showed less excessive bleeding with active management but more adverse effects such as; increased incidence of raised blood pressure, nausea and vomiting. Interestingly, it also showed much lower incidences of excessive bleeding in the physiological arm of the trial than in the Bristol study, though it is always difficult to compare data between different trials. There were more retained placentas (and therefore manual removals of placentas) in the group of women who had actively managed third stages of labour.

In the smaller Brighton trial (Thiliganathan et al 1993), the main findings were that there was no difference in blood loss between the groups of women having physiological or active management of the third stage. More significantly, haemoglobin levels were similar in the two groups of women three days after birth. The third stage of labour in this trial was found to be longer in the group of women who had a physiological third stage. The recent Cochrane Review, however, has cautioned that the findings of this trial might not be reliable (Begley et al 2010).

The Hinchingbrooke Trial

Based on their own practice and a desire for better knowledge (see Gyte 1994), researchers carried out the Hinchingbrooke trial (Rogers & Wood 1998). This trial was unusual in that it took place in a hospital where physiological third stage was more common. However, in questionnaires completed by 92 of the 153 midwives involved in the trial, 84% of them said that they felt 'very confident' in active management, but only 42% of them said that they felt 'very confident' in expectant management (Begley et al 2010, p22).

The trial showed that the rate of blood loss over 500 mls was two and a half times greater in women who had a physiological third stage (16.5%) compared with women who had active management (6.8%). Blood loss over 1000mls was 2.6% in the women who had physiological third stages and 1.7% in women who had active management: this was not statistically significant. There was no difference in the number of retained placentas. The results of the trial also further confirmed the side-effects of Syntometrine. Women who had physiological third stages had slightly heavier babies, and it was thought that this was probably because of the extra blood they received while the cord was still pulsating after birth (Rogers et al 1998, Rogers & Wood 1999).

Subsequent Research

Since the first edition of this booklet was published, a number of other studies and trials have been published within scientific and medical journals. Most of these, however, have continued to focus on which drug should be used and the timing, amount and route of administration. Given that this places the focus firmly on how active management should be conducted, their findings are not particularly helpful for women and midwives who want to know about the relative merits of different approaches. Some of these were trials either to compare active and mixed management or different forms of active management (Gülmezoglu et al 2009, Jerbi et al 2007, Hoffman et al 2006, Vasegh et al 2005, Ramirez et al 2001, Khan et al 1997) while others have not been published fully and are thus currently unavailable (see, for example, Muller 1996).

We found one recent randomised controlled trial that purported to compare actively managed and physiological third stage. This study (Kashanian et al 2010) was carried out in Iran, but the women who had so-called expectant management were given an oxytocic (10mg of oxytocin in 500ml of normal saline, administered intravenously) after the birth of the placenta. This is not physiological third stage (see Wickham 2010) and is thus not helpful in this debate.

Systematic Reviews

The most recent systematic review in this area was published by the Cochrane Collaboration in 2010 (Begley et al 2010). Cecily Begley and her colleagues included the four trials mentioned above that compared active management and physiological third stage (Rogers and Wood 1999, Prendeville and Elbourne 1998, Thiliganathan et al 1993, Begley 1990a, 1990b) plus another that compared active management with mixed management (Khan et al 1997) and concluded that:

'Active management of third stage reduced the risk of haemorrhage greater than 1000ml in an unselected population, but adverse effects

are identified. Women should be given information on the benefits and harms to support informed choice. Given the concerns about early cord clamping and the potential adverse effects of some uterotonics, it is critical now to look at the individual components of third stage management. Data are also required from low-income countries.' (Begley et al 2010: 2).

This Review is significantly different from the previous Review (Prendiville 2000) and is important for a number of reasons:

1. The authors point out that the trials they examined all took place in hospital where active management was the norm, and that this may impact on findings. They acknowledge the limitations of the research on which conclusions about third stage management have been based, and the uncertainties about which women may benefit from expectant or active management, and which components of these may be beneficial or harmful.

2. They suggest that women at low risk of bleeding may suffer from raised blood pressure, after pains requiring analgesics and secondary bleeding, without a reduction in severe bleeding after birth. However, the specific choice of uterotonic may show differences here. The review suggests that women at low risk of bleeding may benefit from expectant third stage management and that they should only receive active management in the event of actual bleeding.

3. The authors note that the reduction in blood loss in the population of birthing women in high income countries, irrespective of risk of bleeding, is an average reduction. *'Thus it may not necessarily be true that all methods of active management will have the reported size of advantages in terms of*

PPH [postpartum haemorrhage], *or other outcomes, over all methods of expectant management.'* (Begley et al 2010, p24).

4. They point out that in one study the mean blood loss among the group of women who had active management was more than in the group of women who had expectant management in another study.

5. The review also acknowledges that babies have lower birth weights following active management. It attributes this to reduced blood volume following early cord clamping, and acknowledges that this could compromise babies by causing anaemia which might impact on their long term health and development.

At the time of writing, this review is freely available online from the Cochrane Library (www.cochrane.org).

Chapter 5

Wider Issues

This chapter deals with a number of wider issues around placental birth, including uncertainties, questions that need to be researched, notes on specific situations and other thinking on this subject.

The Limitations of Existing Research

In the previous chapter we discussed the research trials that have been carried out on third stage management as well as the most recent systematic review which has examined these trials. One significant issue relates to the limitations of these research studies, which include that:

- The way that physiological third stage was defined in these trials, the environment within which it took place and the practices which were associated with it may be different from the way that some experienced midwives would facilitate a physiological placental birth in a woman's home or in midwife run birth centres, so the results do not necessarily apply in these settings. They may also not apply where experienced midwives facilitate a physiological third stage in hospital, and we discuss this further in the section on setting and practitioner expertise on page 74.

- An interesting and related criticism of the randomised controlled trials to date is that, in all groups in the trials, the third stage is in fact 'managed' (Odent 1998b). Michel Odent (2002, 1998b), Kathleen Fahy (2009) and others suggest that expectant third stage management is defined in negative terms in relation to active management, i.e. it is an avoidance of active management. It has not been defined in positive terms, i.e. factors that may promote the safety and efficiency of a natural third stage. They believe that the research is therefore biased towards managed third stage from the outset and that disturbances to the physiological processes have a major influence on the third stage. They claim that in the randomised trials to date, physiological processes are *'highly disturbed both in the study groups and the control groups.'* (Odent 1998b).

- All of the research has been based around the quantitative measurement of blood loss. As we mentioned above, some women can lose more blood than others without being compromised, and it is important to look at other measures of wellbeing. New Zealand midwife Kirsty Prichard, along with others, suggests that *'an assessment of the woman's physiological response to the blood loss'* be considered (Prichard et al 1995, p10).

- Many of the women who were in the 'physiological third stage' group in the trials experienced elements of active management – also known as 'mixed management' – so, again, physiological placental birth has not really been studied within these trials. The studies that we have tell us that active management would appear to be preferable to a mixture of mixed management and physiological placental birth. This information, however, is not helpful for those who want to know about the effectiveness and safety of physiological placental birth or who want to look at different kinds of mixed management.

- In some of the studies, women who were in the physiological third stage group experienced other interventions in labour which are known to increase the likelihood of bleeding and which some experienced midwives see as a contraindication to physiological placental birth (or at least would not be surprised to see a greater than average blood loss). Even if the women in the physiological third stage groups had all experienced physiological placental birth, the inclusion of women who experienced these other interventions (which include having certain drugs for pain relief in labour or having an episiotomy) means that physiological placental birth was not properly evaluated.

- There was wide variation in the practices which constituted both types of 'management' which, as Begley et al (2010) noted, makes it difficult to compare the studies and to use the pooled data (the combined results of several studies) to come to meaningful conclusions. Because of this, not all forms of active management will have the advantages that the overall pooled data suggest, and there is thus a need for caution as well as further research.

- None of the research considered psychophysiological outcomes for mothers and babies. Sarah Buckley (2011) suggests that physiological placenta birth could benefit women and their babies in terms of the immediate and ongoing interaction between them through bonding, breastfeeding and well-being.

Adaptations and Questions Arising from the Research

Because there is such an overlap between active and expectant third stage management, midwife Louise Long (2003) suggests using the term 'adaptive care'. This may be a useful term to help us to better understand that these categories are not absolute. It may also help us to identify the individual components of active management to see which of these are more or less effective if women want, or need, the birth of their placenta to be actively managed. This is also suggested by the Cochrane Review (Begley et al 2010).

Many people, including Begley et al (2010), have highlighted evidence to show that women who have had active management are more likely to return to hospital after they have gone home due to bleeding. This can be because a part of their placenta has remained in their uterus and they go on to have excessive bleeding during the first few days after birth (secondary bleeding). While we do not yet have research evidence that looks at this in detail, some people believe that the retention of part of the placenta might be caused by the controlled cord traction, where the midwife pulls the placenta to get it out before the oxytocic drug acts to fully contract the uterus. Begley et al (2010) suggest that we need to examine whether if a woman is bleeding or is at high risk of bleeding, it would be as effective to give her a uterotonic after the cord has stopped pulsating and been clamped. While this practice is being carried out in some areas (and is an example of the 'adaptive care' that Louise Long discussed), we have no data considering its effectiveness.

The Cochrane Review (Begley et al 2010) also strongly suggests that:

- All further research should look at *'maternal, fetal and infant outcomes.'* (p25).

- We should consider whether women at low risk of bleeding should be offered physiological third stage and only given treatment for active bleeding. NICE (2007) suggests that this should happen if women request it.

- Raised blood pressure, after pains and secondary bleeding be examined.

- We look at how we can minimise the potential harms of active management.

- Researchers determine what reduces blood loss, and whether a uterotonic on its own (i.e. without other elements such as cord clamping and cutting and controlled cord traction) has this effect.

The authors of the Review finally suggest that women at low risk of bleeding should be included in studies about expectant management. They suggest that different aspects of this should be considered, for example, the mother actively pushing her placenta out, with or without gentle cord traction, or giving a uterotonic after expectant management (though experienced midwives suggest that this causes severe after pains, as well as vomiting if Ergometrine is used). The authors of the Review also suggest that studies on active management should include women at risk of bleeding and compare different forms of active management.

Kathleen Fahy (2009) questions whether or not a randomised controlled trial could be done on third stage management, because women should only be randomised after the birth of the baby as it is only at this point that it is clear whether or not a woman has had a normal labour and birth and is at low risk of bleeding. She suggests that it would be unethical to randomise women at this stage of labour. Other researchers believe that randomisation should happen as close to the intervention as possible, and that this could occur just before the birth of the baby, as long as the woman has full information during pregnancy and gives consent again during labour. These researchers acknowledge the ethical difficulties of informed consent, but argue that we need to balance arguments against carrying out a randomised controlled trial in the context that without them, clinicians will do what they believe to be best – in this case active management of the third stage of labour (Gill Gyte 2010 personal communication). Some experienced midwives and others studying physiology have expressed concern that asking women to think about different third stage approaches and give consent during this crucial phase of labour might in itself be an intervention and impact on delicate hormonal changes and thus the birth process.

Exploring Other Ways of Knowing

One of the problems with basing practice purely on scientific research, especially randomised controlled trials, is that it can disregard crucial experiential and observational knowledge. Well-designed and expertly carried out research trials can give us good information about treatments and practices involving large groups of people, but tell us little about individuals – the differences between people and the subtle affects of treatments and procedures. Experiential and observational knowledge often provides the basis for more systematic research, but also tells us about individuals and practices which may be less easily measured by quantitative, scientific research.

For example, some experienced midwives in Britain and other countries do not recommend the routine use of Syntometrine or Syntocinon for the third stage of labour, but suggest that these should be used only when needed. They do, however, emphasise the need to develop an ongoing relationship with women, so that among other issues, they can consider the likelihood of the woman bleeding after birth and can take steps in pregnancy to reduce any risks – possibly through dietary or lifestyle changes. There is a need to acknowledge the importance of continuity of carer and the development of mutual understanding so that the woman and midwife can work together during labour and birth to optimise the likelihood of all going well. In addition, in the unlikely event of bleeding occurring unexpectedly, this trust enables them to work together efficiently and deal with the emergency as safely and quickly as possible.

Midwives practising this way rely on scientific evidence to guide their practice. However, they also use their own experiential knowledge, and that of others, which has usually been gained over many years. While they expect birth to unfold safely, they are alert at all times to the possibility of unexpected changes, which may require rapid and efficient responses. They also heed their intuition, and because the relationship with the woman is central to their practice, they are attuned to the women in their care.

One midwife described an unusual incident of a woman having a velamentous insertion of the cord (where the vessels of the cord separate and go through the membranes before reaching the placenta). The midwife knew the woman, had been with her during two previous births, knew that the pattern of her labour was unusual for her and encouraged her to follow her instincts despite the unusually slow, stop-start progress of her labour. The midwife was reminded of Australian GP, John Stevenson's observation that this can be a sign of the body taking care of a problem with the cord – such as a knot. The midwife refrained from intervening with the normal course of labour and the baby was born healthy and well. Only after the arrival of the placenta was the midwife able to understand the problem. It is possible that any of the standard medical interventions for a 'prolonged' labour could have seriously compromised the baby and may even have been fatal (Wolford 1997). While we need to be cautious of anecdotal experiences, these can sometimes provide pointers when put alongside other evidence.

It seems we still have some way to go in balancing different forms of knowledge, and have much to learn from midwives and doctors who have incorporated openness to different ways of knowing in their own practices and who listen to women, observe carefully, and treat each woman as an individual.

The Impact of Setting and Practitioner Expertise

We have already mentioned that all of the research trials making comparisons between different ways of managing the third stage of labour have been carried out in hospitals, and that some people believe that the setting and environment may be an important factor in the outcome of the birth of the placenta. A study in New Zealand (Prichard et al 1995) which looked at 213 women who had home births lent support to this argument. The emphasis was on the lack of disturbance to the physiological processes of birth, and showed that 3.3% of the women had postpartum haemorrhages (defined as a blood loss over 500mls). None of the women required a manual removal of the placenta. Interestingly, the lengths of the first, second and third stages of labour bore no relation to blood loss. There was a tendency for women with higher haemoglobin counts in late pregnancy (possibly indicating less than optimum haemodilution) to lose more blood after birth, and 15% of the women who had had previous postpartum haemorrhages had a subsequent one. Crucially, no woman had a reported blood loss of more than 900ml. However, the researchers acknowledged that estimated blood loss can be inaccurate and that the methods used in this research may have introduced bias. They concluded that it raised important issues for exploration rather than providing definitive answers.

A worrying factor which came to light in a research study (Logue 1990) was the impact of the individual practitioner on the occurrence of postpartum haemorrhage. It was discovered that, in one particular hospital, the postpartum haemorrhage rates varied from 1-16% for midwives, and 1-31% for registrars. Doctors and midwives considered to be 'heavy-handed', had much higher rates. No subsequent research has been carried out, despite the fact that this seems to be an important finding.

More recent analyses discussed in the Cochrane Review (Begley et al 2010) suggest that the skill of the practitioner is a crucial factor in supporting physiological third stage. The review cites observational studies in Holland and New Zealand where midwives may be more skilled in physiological placental birth than in some other areas. These showed that there was no reduction in blood loss among the women who had their third stages actively managed. In the New Zealand study, 33,752 women were included. All had had physiological labours and births. Almost a half of these women had physiological third stages and their blood loss was slightly less than the women who had active management of the third stage of labour (Begley et al 2010).

A very recent addition to the literature on placental birth comes from Australia (Fahy et al 2010). This retrospective cohort study (looking at the outcomes of births that have already happened) carried out by Kathleen Fahy, Carolyn Hastie and colleagues included 3436 women who were at low risk of postpartum haemorrhage, who had had no interventions during labour and birth and had no predisposing factors. 3075 of these women gave birth in a tertiary unit (usually a large obstetric unit) and 361 of these women gave birth in free standing midwifery unit. The researchers compared 'holistic psychophysioloical care' with active management of the third stage of labour. The 'holistic psychophysiological' care was described in contrast to the usual 'expectant care', and included creating a conducive environment in which the woman feels:

'safe, secure, cared about and trusting that her privacy is respected. The attending midwife must be knowledgeable and feel confident about optimising psychophysiology during the third stage of labour.' (p147-148).

This includes:

'immediate and sustained skin-to-skin contact between the woman and the baby who are both kept warm; the midwife gently encourages the woman to focus on her baby whilst maintaining awareness that the placenta is yet to be born; the support people remain focused on mother and baby; there is "self-attachment" breastfeeding; the midwife unobtrusively observes for signs of separation of the placenta; there is no fundal massage or meddling; the placenta is birthed entirely by maternal effort and gravity. The midwife or the woman gently "checks the fundus" for 1 hour postplacental birth to ensure contraction and haemostasis.' [stopping of bleeding] (p148).

Of the women who were at low risk of bleeding too much after birth, 3075 gave birth in the tertiary unit and most received active management. 344 of these women had blood losses over 500mls (11.2%). The 361 women who had their babies in the free standing midwifery led unit mostly had 'psychophysiological' care and 10 of them had blood losses of over 500ml (2.8%). Taking the two units together showed that of the 3016 women who had active management, 347 had blood losses of over 500mls (11.5%) and of the 420 women who received psychophysiological care 7 had blood losses of over 500mls (1.7%). The number of women who had blood losses of over 1000, or 1500mls was extremely small, but was slightly higher in those women who had active management in the tertiary unit. The researchers concluded that holistic psychophysiological care for the third stage of labour is safe for women who are at low risk of bleeding excessively after birth. While the researchers acknowledge that there are limitations to their study and suggest more research needs to be done, the results are not altogether surprising and begin to address the call by the Cochrane Review authors (Begley et al 2010) that women at low risk of bleeding excessively after birth need to be considered separately in further trials (see Essentially MIDIRS (2011) for further comment on Fahy et al's study).

AIMS - Association for Improvements in Maternity Services

A NOTE ABOUT WATERBIRTH

We have observed that there is some variation in the practices around the birth of women's placentas where they have given birth to their baby in water. In some areas, even though the policy in most hospitals is to recommend managed third stage (sometimes quite strongly), women who give birth in water are told that they will need to have a physiological placental birth. It is not clear why this is, although it may be a consequence of the myth that waterbirth is associated with a hypothetical risk of water embolism (see Wickham 2005) and/or because midwives are not easily able to administer an oxytocic and/or perform the manoeuvres associated with active management while women remain in the pool.

In most maternity units in the UK, it is policy for women to be asked to leave the pool before the birth of their placenta. There are various factors influencing such policies, for example, concerns about not being able to measure blood loss (though experienced midwives suggest that this is possible), and not being able to get a woman out of the pool quickly enough in the case of an emergency. The level of concern depends on the midwife's knowledge, skill and confidence, and these concerns may be exacerbated when women and midwives do not know each other before labour.

> We can find no evidence to support a policy of requiring a woman to leave the pool for the birth of the placenta. The usual practice of midwives who are experienced at facilitating physiological placental birth is to follow the woman's lead as far as staying in or getting out of the pool is concerned, unless she appears to be bleeding more than usual. The midwife might then ask her to get out of the pool in order to better assess, and, if necessary, treat this. Any interruption for no reason, at this delicate time, may disrupt the birth of the placenta and should be avoided unless necessary.

Thinking Physiology

Some midwives believe that by considering the theory and their experience of physiology, we could gain a better understanding of issues which currently lack good research evidence. One of us (Sara) described how, when she briefly worked on a hospital postnatal ward after having been a home birth midwife experienced in attending women having natural placental birth, she noticed that the women who had had actively managed third stages often lost large clots when they first visited the toilet 2-3 hours after having given birth.

> *'I realised that their blood loss was probably more noticeable to me because I had previously been practising in a situation in which the majority of women chose physiological third stage. After a physiological third stage, the women did not have the pattern of heavy bleeding delayed for a few hours after the birth that I was observing in the women who had had active management in the hospital. It struck me that this might account for the different*

amounts of blood lost between women who had physiological and managed third stage. Could the use of an oxytocic inhibit the normal blood loss at birth, but cause the blood to be somehow retained by the woman's body and expelled later? This would account both for the difference in recorded blood loss at birth and the later loss of blood in women experiencing active management. Physiologically, this would make sense. The use of an oxytocic drug causes a strong and sustained contraction of the uterus. The uterus is too well contracted to release a large amount of blood at this stage, which is why the blood loss is smaller in most cases.' (Wickham 1999, p14).

The article quoted above also questioned whether or not it is preferable to minimise blood loss given that it may be normal physiology for some women to lose more blood than others, and because a woman's blood volume increases during pregnancy. Blood loss after birth is part of the return to normal physiology:

'[I]f the woman's body is physiologically adapted to losing more blood, it wouldn't be until the effects of the oxytocic had started to wear off that the uterus would be able to relax sufficiently to achieve this. So it may be that the average amount of blood lost during physiological third stage is "normal", while the lesser amounts of blood lost during active management are abnormally low. If we recorded the amount of lochia [blood] lost in the first few hours after birth together with that lost during the birth itself, would the figures for the two types of third stage correlate more closely? Could it be that the total blood loss in women experiencing active management might actually be higher?' (Wickham 1999, p15).

As above, the theory that active management may lead to more blood loss than is counted in the research trials is supported by the findings of Begley et al (2010) who cite the increased likelihood of women who have experienced active management returning to the hospital in the postnatal period. Again, it may be interesting to note that, until Begley et al's (2010) updated Cochrane Review, the standard definition of a postpartum haemorrhage was 500ml, which is the same volume of blood that is taken during blood donation, after which people are offered a cup of tea and a biscuit rather than being considered to have had a haemorrhage!

Another current theory which needs to be researched suggests that pharmaceutical use of oxytocin may reduce a woman's ability to produce her own natural oxytocin in subsequent labours and births.

LOTUS BIRTH

Lotus birth *'is the practice of leaving the umbilical cord uncut, so that the baby remains attached to his or her placenta until the cord naturally separates at the umbilicus, exactly as a cut cord does, at three to ten days after birth.'* (Buckley 2005, p40). Women who have experienced lotus birth often report that the cord separates more quickly following lotus birth than when the cord is clamped and cut and a small stump is left to fall off after a few days.

While there appear to be no early written records about the practice of lotus birth, it is practised among some aboriginal peoples. It has also been documented in observations of chimpanzees, but the first written account among humans may be in 1974, when Clair Lotus Day from California, North America decided to leave her baby's cord attached to her baby and placenta until it separated by itself. Hence, Lotus Birth (Buckley 2005).

AIMS - Association for Improvements in Maternity Services

Lotus Birth has been promoted by some mothers, birth activists and educators, and midwives as a *'logical extension of natural childbirth and invites us to reclaim the so-called third stage of labour for our babies and ourselves, and to honour the placenta, our babies' first source of nourishment'* (Buckley 2005, p41).

Benefits are believed to include a slower and gentler transition for the baby into life outside its mother's womb, a time of rest and seclusion for the mother and her baby and immediate family, because if the baby and placenta remain attached, the mother is more likely to stay at home, an acknowledgement of the spiritual aspects of birth and the placenta and a reduction in infection of the cord (Buckley 2005). Lotus Birth is more often practised at home births, but there is no reason why women should not keep baby, cord and placenta intact and together wherever they give birth and lotus birth has been known to occur after a planned caesarean birth (Davies 2007).

Numbers of accounts recommend how best to look after the cord and placenta during the time they remain attached to the baby. Some suggest wiping or washing the placenta after birth, then liberally salting the placenta and adding drops of lavender or some other antiseptic, pleasant herbal preparation. Some suggest keeping the placenta dry and in a bowl or sieve and exposed to air without adding salt, others suggest putting the placenta in a cloth bag and wrapping baby and placenta in a shawl. The placenta has been described as developing a musky smell by some. The

> cord, like the placenta, gradually dries and shrivels, and the cord usually hardens and then separates. Many of these accounts also provide tips on how to handle the baby while still attached to its cord and placenta. (Buckley 2005, Zenack 1998, also see resources list).
>
> One reported comment made by Michel Odent was that lotus birth *'usefully reverses the cultural conditioning that cutting the cord is physiologically necessary.'* (Davis 2010, p177).

Women, Birth and Time

In debates on the third stage once again we are involved in an argument where the natural physiological processes that a woman's body has evolved to experience are pitted against the amount of time that she spends in labour (or, perhaps more cynically, taking up the space of a hospital bed). Who defines 'normal' time for natural processes and who controls it? This is illustrated in a social study of midwifery: *'Even Syntometrine was said to be used in the third stage of labour "to shorten the third stage" as if there was some urgency to end this undesirable condition.'* (Hunt and Symonds, 1995). Later the authors refer to the speed with which women are 'washed and warded' after delivery: *'The staff have been very efficient but perhaps they were not effective. The urgency to complete the process had overtaken everything else.'* Defining retained placenta in terms of time limits may also be misleading (Prichard et al 1995). In healthy women, redefining postpartum haemorrhage as a blood loss of over 1000mls (as suggested by the World Health Organisation) and extending or removing time limits from the third stage of labour, would considerably alter the interpretation of research results to date. The extension or removal of arbitrary time limits would also alter research design in the future. Many midwives, and others, argue that postpartum haemorrhage should be redefined to mean any blood loss that adversely affects a woman's health, rather than a specific amount. Such a definition would further alter research design and results.

It can be argued that the research to date shows only that in a busy maternity unit, where a woman is unlikely to be completely undisturbed during childbirth, (due to time limits and midwives being more familiar with active management), routinely recommending active management of the third stage of labour reduces blood loss after birth and may thus be preferable to many women. This raises many questions and ethical issues about the management of birth in Britain and elsewhere, and whether and how women can be supported to experience physiological births in large obstetric units

It is certain that any significant shift towards physiological placental birth would need to include supporting midwives to gain the knowledge, skills and experience necessary for them to be able to confidently and competently do this. A number of issues would also need to be addressed, including changing protocols to remove the time pressure on birth of the placenta and increasing understanding of practices which interfere with physiology.

But what do women want? At Hinchingbrooke Hospital, where one of the third stage trials was carried out, the researchers commented that *'when physiological management is offered to women as a reasonable option, many will choose it.'* (Rogers and Wood 1999). Of the women who could have taken part in the study, some declined:

504 of these women chose physiological management and 385 chose active management (Rogers et al 1998).

How a Woman Feels During Placental Birth

While defining labour in terms of different stages may be helpful in some ways, there is a danger that we can lose sight of the journey of birth as a whole and apply principles out of context, failing to recognise how the whole process is inter-related.

The way in which a birth unfolds has direct and indirect physical and emotional implications for the relationship between a mother and her baby, and can affect how the mother feels about herself for a long time afterwards. This is as true during the birth of the placenta as it is during any phase of birth. It can be a particularly delicate and awesome time, as the mother sees her baby for the first time and, if all is well, is able slowly to come to terms with becoming a mother and getting to know her baby. Whether the woman and her attendants have decided to await the birth of the placenta by natural means or manage the third stage actively, the atmosphere remains crucial to hormonal balances which impact upon the relationships between the woman, her baby and their family.

A calm, unhurried environment will encourage the mother to get to know her baby in her own time and in her own way. She may want to pick her baby up and put it to her breast, or let the baby begin to take in his/her surroundings, and gaze into her eyes. Whilst the term 'bonding' may have become a cliché, the concept is vital in promoting a healthy start to parenting. It is an ongoing process and is highly significant around the time of birth. Any approach should therefore seek to minimise interference at this time and ideally promote the skin-to-skin contact which we now know is a crucial element of this journey (Hastie 2011, Schmid 2005).

For some women it is important to allow the birth of their placenta to unfold in its own time and to have a sense of completion, relief and triumph, while at the same time changing their focus to the baby.

> 'how wonderful it is when your placenta comes out because it's all soft and not painful. It's actually quite a feeling of relief because it's all squishy and soft ... it is a really nice feeling.'

> 'I felt it like a first kiss with your favourite boyfriend. That sort of mmm in your belly feeling. That's how it was for me. It was like, ping, big electric thing then I just felt it slide out. It was like wow, and it felt lovely.'

For some, the birth of the placenta may be quick and easy, taking minutes, for others it may take a good deal longer. Very occasionally the woman may feel physical discomfort or pain which can be intense and distressing. Some women may still feel over-awed by the birth or feel exhausted, cold, shivery, detached or confused, whilst others are keen to 'get it over with', feeling tired and anxious to put the birth behind them so as to be able to focus on their newborn baby.

There is no 'right' way to give birth but there should be a clear and good reason for any intervention that is suggested, as no intervention is without risk. Good communication between the mother and her attendant is an important component for the mother and the baby's well-being and, whilst controversy surrounds management of the birth of the placenta, it is particularly important that a mutual understanding exists (see Green et al, 1998). In asking the question 'what is the "best" care', policy-makers and caregivers should accept that part of the answer lies in providing individualised care for individual women based on their preferences and individual circumstances. This is more and more difficult in our culture of standardised care, rules and apportioning blame to midwives and parents who break these rules. We invite any woman who wants to discuss aspects of her care to get in touch with AIMS by any of the means listed on page 95.

Placental Birth: Women and Decision Making

Given the inconclusive results and varied interpretation of scientific research and other knowledge and discussion in this area, how can the individual woman make an informed decision about accepting active management of the third stage of labour, or planning for a physiological placental birth? Four important considerations seem to be:

1. The variations in midwives' and doctors' ideology and practices around birth. These might be more aligned with holistic care that supports undisturbed birth where possible, or may be more aligned to an obstetric approach that is more likely to try to control the birth process. These ideologies and practices will extend to the birth of the woman's placenta.

2. The lack of knowledge, skill and experience among health practitioners to help women to birth their placentas physiologically. In recent research, Diane Farrar and her colleagues found that 93% of doctors and 73% of midwives in the UK 'always or usually' use active management of the third stage of labour (Farrar et al 2010).

3. The fact that it can be difficult to identify women at risk of developing problems during this phase of birth with any accuracy – though it seems clear from the Cochrane Review (Begley et al 2010) that women who are healthy, have had normal labours and births and who are at low risk of bleeding excessively benefit from having a natural placental birth by avoiding some of the problems associated with active management.

4. How best to make information available to women to enable them to make their own decisions. Although the National Institute for Clinical Excellence (NICE) still recommends offering active management to women and supports early cord clamping, it also explicitly acknowledges that women with normal pregnancies and births should be supported to have expectant management of the third stage if they wish (NICE 2007). The Cochrane Review suggests that women should be informed about the benefits and harms of active management, and that their decisions should be supported (Begley et al 2010).

There are conditions and circumstances that might increase the likelihood of bleeding after birth. These are often listed in midwifery books, in research papers and elsewhere. Sometimes these lists are extensive, but most are neither definitive nor even necessarily supported by evidence. They might, for example, include:

- known blood clotting disorders – women who bruise or bleed easily or who have particularly heavy periods should be offered testing antenatally and active management may be recommended (Gill Gyte 2010, personal communication).

- antepartum haemorrhage (bleeding during pregnancy).

- third stage problems in a previous labour (but it is important to bear in mind that these may have been caused by inappropriate intervention and women may wish to discuss their experiences with an experienced midwife).
- anaemia.
- expecting more than one baby (a multiple birth).
- a long (prolonged) labour.
- a very fast (precipitate) labour.
- oxytocic drugs during labour – if the woman's labour has been induced or accelerated with an oxytocic drip, the drip will normally be left in place until after the placenta is born.

None of the conditions listed above would automatically cause problems. However, in some of these situations, most midwives would recommend active management. It is essential that when a woman intends to avoid the use of oxytocic drugs and/or other interventions she is able to discuss this fully with a midwife who is knowledgeable and confident about this preference. Women have the right to make their own decisions whatever the circumstances; this issue is covered more extensively in the AIMS booklet 'Am I Allowed?' (Beech 2003).

Research shows that women often know little about the birth of the placenta (Green et al 1998). This point was specifically mentioned by Cecily Begley and her colleagues (2010). They noted that women are now asking their midwives more questions about the birth of their placenta. As the issues are complex, each woman should be able to talk about the third stage with a midwife and receive as much information as possible during her pregnancy. Women should not be expected to consider the pros and cons of physiological placental birth and actively managed third stage for the first time during labour or after the baby's birth. Neither should women be asked to tick a box during pregnancy expressing their preference without having been given information upon which to base this decision.

Women should receive detailed information about both the benefits and harms of different approaches to placental birth, and that healthy women at low risk of bleeding too much after birth, following actively managed third stage, are more likely to have raised blood pressure, after pains and secondary bleeding, without a reduction in severe bleeding. They should also know that they can receive active management as a treatment if it becomes necessary and that this will be as effective as prophylactic active management. Women who are more likely to bleed too much after birth, or who prefer active management should be aware of the potential benefits of delayed cord clamping for their babies, and that syntocinon, for example, may be as effective as syntometrine without causing raised blood pressure.

A Final Word

Women use information and interpret research in different ways, and their personal values and beliefs will affect their decisions. They should always be respected and supported. This issue is and will continue to be problematic if midwives are expected to follow national and/or local policies that recommend routine active management of the third stage of labour at the same time as their professional rules and guidance and personal integrity emphasise the importance of providing woman-centred care.

Post Script

A few days before this booklet went to press, a research study (Grotegut et al 2011) was published which was very relevant to the content of this booklet. We have included it here because we believe the findings are significant and add to the debate herein.

The study looked at women who had experienced excessive bleeding which was related to their uterus not contracting well after the birth. The researchers compared the amounts of oxytocin that had been given to women during labour, who had excessive bleeding after birth and the amount given to women who had not experienced excessive bleeding after birth, but who were similar in other ways. The results showed that the women who had excessive bleeding had been given more than two and a half times the amount of oxytocin during labour than the other women. The researchers carried out a number of statistical tests which indicated that this was not due to other differences such as induction of labour, body mass index (BMI) or race.

We believe that this is significant because when women are given substantial amounts of oxytocin during labour, this has a detrimental effect on the ability of their uterine muscle to effectively contract after birth.

AIMS - Association for Improvements in Maternity Services

Chapter 6

Resources and References

Further Reading

Buckley S (2009) *Gentle Birth, Gentle Mothering.* Berkeley, CA: Celestial Arts.

Beech BAL (2003) *Am I Allowed? Yes, Yes, Yes.* London: AIMS.

Enkin M, Kierse MJNC, Nielson J et al (2000) *A Guide to Effective Care in Pregnancy and Childbirth, Third Edition,* Oxford University Press.

Gurnsey J, Davies S (2010) A care pathway for the physiological third stage of labour. *Essentially MIDIRS,* 1 (4), 32-36.

Inch S (1989) *Birthrights.* London: Greenprint.

Mercer JS, Nelson CC, Skovgaard RL (2000) Umbilical cord clamping: beliefs and practices of American nurse-midwives. *Journal of Midwifery & Women's Health 2000*; 45(1), 58–66.

Mercer JS (2001) Current best evidence: a review of the literature on umbilical cord clamping. *Journal of Midwifery & Women's Health 2001*; 46(6), 402–14.

Mercer JS, Skovgaard R, Erickson-Owens D (2008) Fetal to neonatal transition: first do no harm. *In:* Downe S, ed. *Normal Childbirth: evidence and debate.* 2nd Edition. Edinburgh: Churchill Livingstone, 2008, 149–74.

Mercer J; Erikson-Owens D (2010) Evidence for neonatal transition and the first hour of life. *In*: Walsh D, Downe S, eds. (2010) *Essential midwifery practice: intrapartum care*. Chichester: John Wiley, 81-104.

Priya JV (1992) *Birth Traditions and Modern Pregnancy Care*. Rockport MA: Element.

A National Childbirth Trust information page on the Third Stage of Labour is available from www.nctpregnancyandbabycare.com

Useful websites

www.aims.org.uk

www.birthspirit.co.nz

www.homebirth.org.uk/thirdstage.htm

www.midwifery.org.uk

www.midwiferytoday.com

www.nct.org.uk/info-centre/decisions/view-92

www.sarahjbuckley.com

www.thirdstageoflabour.org.uk

www.withwoman.co.uk

Lotus Birth

www.joyousbirth.info/articles/lotus-birth.html

www.sarahjbuckley.com/articles/lotus-birth.htm

www.lotusfertility.com/The_Spiritual_Principles_of_Lotus_Birth.html

www.lotusfertility.com/Lotus_Birth_For_Midwives.html

en.wikipedia.org/wiki/Lotus_birth

www.caesarean.org.uk/birthReports/WandaCS.html

More Information

AIMS
Beverley Lawrence Beech, 5 Ann's Court, Grove Road, Surbiton, Surrey, KT6 4BE
0300 365 0663
helpline@aims.org.uk
www.aims.org.uk

Our publications list is available on our website www.aims.org.uk

MIDIRS (Midwives Information and Research Service)
9 Elmdale Road Clifton, Bristol B58 1SL Tel: 0117 925 1791
www.midirs.org

NCT
Alexandra House, Oldham Terrace, London W3 6NH
Tel: 0181 992 8637
www.nct.org.uk

References

Anderson T (1998) Prophylactic syntometrine vs oxytocin in the third stage of labour. *Practising Midwife*, Vol 1, No 10, 40-41.

Anderson T (1999) Active versus expectant management of the third stage of labour. *Practising Midwife*, Vol 2, No 2, 10-11.

Baskett TF (2000) A flux of reds: evolution of active management of the third stage of labour. *Journal of the Royal Society of Medicine*, Vol 93, No 3, 489-493.

Beech BL, Robinson J (1994) *Ultrasound Unsound.* London: AIMS.

Begley CM (1990a) A comparison of 'active' and 'physiological' management of the third stage of labour. *Midwifery*, Vol 6, No 1, 3-17.

Begley CM (1990b) The effect of ergometrine on breastfeeding. *Midwifery*, Vol 6, No 2, 60-72.

Begley CM, Gyte GM, Murphy DJ, Devane D, McDonald SJ, McGuire W (2010) Active versus expectant management for women in the third stage of labour. *Cochrane Database of Systematic Reviews* Issue 7: http://www.thecochranelibrary.com.

Beech BL (2003) *Am I Allowed? Yes, Yes, Yes.* London: AIMS.

Bloomfield TH, Gordon H (1990) Reaction to blood loss at delivery. *Journal of Obstetrics and Gynaecology*, Vol 10 (Suppl 2): S13–S16.

Botha MC (1968) The management of the umbilical cord in labour. *South African Journal of Obstetrics and Gynaecology*, Vol 16, No 2, 30-33.

Buckley S (2011) Ask Away: Are there any psychophysiological benefits to women of physiological third stage management compared with active management of the third stage of labour? *Essentially MIDIRS*, Vol 2, No 3, 37-38.

Buckley S (2009) *Gentle Birth, Gentle Mothering.* Berkeley, CA: Celestial Arts.

Buckley SJ (2005) *Gentle Birth, Gentle Mothering.* Brisbane: One Moon Press.

Burnley M, Roberts CL, Thatcher R, Doust JH, Jones AM (2006) Influence of blood donation on O2 uptake on kinetics, peak O2 uptake and time to exhaustion during severe-intensity cycle exercise in humans. *Experimental Physiology,* Vol 91, 499–509.

Caliskan E, Dilbaz B, Meydanli MM, *et al* (2003) Oral misoprostol for the third stage of labor: a randomized controlled trial. *Obstetrics and Gynecology,* Vol 101, No 5, part 1, 921-928.

Caliskan E, Meydanli M, Dilbaz B, et al (2002) Is rectal misoprostol really effective in the treatment of third stage of labor? A randomized controlled trial. *American Journal of Obstetrics and Gynecology,* Vol 187, No 4, 1038-1045.

Chalmers I (1990) Care during the third stage of labour, Commentary on a Commentary. *AIMS Quarterly Journal*, Vol 2, No 3, 8-11.

Confidential Enquiry into Maternal and Child Health (2009) *Perinatal mortality 2007*: United Kingdom. London: CEMACH.

Choy CMY, Lau WC, Tam WH, and others (2002) A randomised controlled trial of intramuscular syntometrine and intravenous oxytocin in the management of the third stage of labour . *BJOG: An International Journal of Obstetrics and Gynaecology,* Vol 109, No 2, 173-177.

Cook CM, Spurrett B, Murray H (1999) A randomized clinical trial comparing oral misoprostol with synthetic oxytocin or syntometrine in the third stage of labour. *Australian and New Zealand Journal of Obstetrics and Gynaecology,* Vol 39, No 4, 414-419.

Cronk M, Flint C (1989) *Community Midwifery: A Practical Guide.* Heinemann Medical Books. Chapter 4, 50-71.

Cumming DC, Taylor PJ (1978) Puerperal uterine inversion: report of nine cases. *Canadian Medical Association Journal,* Vol 118, No 10, 1268-70.

Darwin E (1801) *Zoonomia: Or the laws of organic life.* Third Edition, London, J Johnson, 32.

Davies L (2007) Would you like a lotus birth with that ma'am? The increasing menu of choice and caesarean section. *MIDIRS Midwifery Digest,* Vol 17, No 4, 463-466.

Davis J (2010) Striking gorilla hormones, compelling circles and awesome plastic bag tricks: experiences of attending the Midatlantic conference on birth and primal health research, Gran Canaria, 26-28 February 2010. *MIDIRS Midwifery Digest,* Vol 20, No 2, 176-178.

Davis-Floyd RE, Barclay L, Daviss BA, and Tritten J (2009) *Birth Models That Work.* University of California Press.

de Groot ANJA, van Roosmalen J, van Dongen PWJ (1996) Survey of the management of third stage of labour in the Netherlands. *European Journal of Obstetrics and Gynaecology and Reproductive Biology,* Vol 66, 39-40.

Department of Health (1998) *Why mothers die: report on confidential enquiries into maternal deaths in the United Kingdom.* 1994-6, London: HMSO.

Dewhurst J (1990) The prevention of postpartum haemorrhage: A Review. *Journal of Obstetrics and Gynaecology,* Vol 10, Suppl 2.

Diab KM, Ramy AR, Yehia MA (1999) The use of rectal misoprostol as active pharmacological management of the third stage of labor. *Journal of Obstetrics and Gynaecology Research,* Vol 25, No 5, 327-332.

Dixon L, Fletcher L, Tracy S, et al (2009) Midwives care during the Third Stage of labour: An analysis of the New Zealand College of Midwives Midwifery Database 2004-2008. *New Zealand College of Midwives Journal,* 41, 20-25.

Dunn PM (2004/5) Clamping the umbilical cord. *AIMS Journal,* Vol 16, No 4, 8-9.

Dunn PM (1991) The third stage of labour and fetal adaptation at birth. Wyeth Guest Lecture, *1st International Congress of Perinatal Medicine,* Tokyo, November 7.

Dunn PM (1989) Perinatal factors influencing adaptation to extrauterine life. Advances in Gynaecology and Obstetrics, Vol 5, *Pregnancy and Labour. Proc. 12th World Congress Obstetrics and. Gynecology*, Rio de Janeiro, Oct. (1988) Ed by Belfort P, Pinotti JA, Eskes TKAB Parthenon Publ, Carnforth, Lancs, Vol 15, 119-123.

Dunn PM (1985) Management of childbirth in normal women. The third stage and fetal adaption. Perinatal medicine. *Proceedings of the IX European Congress Perinatal Medicine,* Dublin, September 1984. MTP Press, Chapter 7, 47-54.

Dunn PM, Frazer ID, Raper AB (1966) Influence of early cord ligation on the transplacental passage of the foetal cells. *Journal of Obstetrics and Gynaecology of the British Commonwealth,* Vol 73, 757-760.

Edmunds J (1998) Hemorrhage: stay close and pay attention to your mothers. *Midwifery Today,* Vol 48, 14-16.

Enkin M, Kierse MJNC, Chalmers I (1991) *A Guide to Effective Care in Pregnancy and Childbirth.* Oxford University Press, Chapter 36.

Enkin M, Kierse MJNC, Nielson J, Renfrew M (1995) *A Guide to Effective Care in Pregnancy and Childbirth.* Second Edition, Oxford University Press.

Essentially MIDIRS (2011) MIDIRS Update: Holistic physiological care compared with active management of the third stage of labour for women at low risk of postpartum haemorrhage: a cohort study. *Essentially MIDIRS,* Vol 2, No 1, 6.

Fadiman A (1997) *The spirit catches you and you fall down - a Hmong child, her American doctors and the collision of two cultures.* New York: Farrar, Straus and Giroux.

Fahy K, Hastie C, Bisits A, Marsh C, Smith L, Saxton A (2010) Holistic physiological care compared to active management of the third stage of labour for women at low risk of postpartum haemorrhage: A cohort study. *Midwifery and Birth,* Vol 23, 146-152.

Fahy KM (2009) Third stage of labour care for women at low risk of postpartum haemorrhage. *Journal of Midwifery and Women's Health,* Vol 54, No 5, 380-386.

Farrar D, Airey R, Low GR, Tuffnell D, Cattle B, Duley L (2011) Measuring placental transfusion for term births: weighing babies with cord intact. *BJOG: An International Journal of Obstetrics and Gynaecology,* Vol 118, 70-75.

Farrar D, Tuffnell D, Airey R and Duley L (2010) Care during the third stage of labour: A postal survey of UK midwives and obstetricians. *BMC Pregnancy and Childbirth 2010,* 10:23 doi:10.1186/1471-2393-10-23.

Featherstone IE (1999) Physiological third stage of labour. *British Journal of Midwifery,* Vol 7, No 4, 216-221.

Fraser DM and Cooper MA (2003) *Myles Textbook for Midwives.* Edinburgh: Churchill Livingstone.

Fraser DM and Cooper MA (2009) *Myles Textbook for Midwives.* Edinburgh: Churchill Livingstone.

Foureur M (2008) Creating birth space to enable undisturbed birth. In: Fahy K, Foureur M, Hastie C, eds. *Birth Territory and Midwifery Guardianship: Theory for Practice. Education and Research.* Edinburgh: Books for Midwives 57-77.

Garg P, Batra S, Gandhi G (2005) Oral misoprostol versus injectable methylergometrine in management of the third stage of labor. *International Journal of Gynecology and Obstetrics,* Vol 91, No 2, 160-161.

Gerstenfeld TS, Wing DA (2001) Rectal misoprostol versus intravenous oxytocin for the prevention of postpartum hemorrhage after vaginal delivery. *American Journal of Obstetrics and Gynecology,* Vol 185I, No 4, 878-882.

Green JM, Coupland VA, Kitzinger JV (1998) *Great expectations: a prospective study of women's expectations and experiences of childbirth.* Cheshire Books for Midwives Press, Vol 2 Chapter 6, 322-347.

Grotegut CA, Paglia MJ, Johnson LNC et al (2011) Oxytocin exposure during labor among women with postpartum hemorrhage secondary to uterine atony. *American Journal of Obstetrics and Gynecology,* Vol 204, No 1 56.e1-6.

Gülmezoglu AM (1998) Prostaglandins for the management for the third stage of labour (Cochrane Review) In: *The Cochrane Library,* Issue 4. Oxford: Update Software.

Gülmezoglu AM, Widmer M, Merialdi M, Qureshi Z, Piaggio G, Elbourne D, et al (2009) Active management of the third stage of labour without controlled cord traction: a randomized noninferiority controlled trial. *Reproductive Health*, Vol 6, No 2 [doi: 10.1186/1742-4755-6-2].

Gülmezoglu AM, Forna F, Villar J, Hofmeyr GJ. Prostaglandins for preventing postpartum haemorrhage. *Cochrane Database of Systematic Reviews 2007*, Issue 3. Art. No.: CD000494. doi: 10.1002/14651858.CD000494.pub3.

Gurnsey J, Davies S (2010) A care pathway for the physiological third stage of labour. *Essentially MIDIRS*, Vol 1, No 4, 32-36.

Gyte G (1998) Informed choice and the third stage of labour. *Research Matters*, No 7. Available from NCT.

Gyte G (1994) Evaluation of the meta-analysis on the effects on both mother and baby, of the various components of 'active management' of the third stage of labour. *Midwifery*, Vol 10, 183-199.

Gyte G (1992) The significance of blood loss at delivery. *MIDIRS Midwifery Digest*, Vol 2, No 1, 88-92.

Gyte G (1991) The continuing debate on the third stage of labour. *AIMS Quarterly Journal*, Vol 3, No 1, 4-6.

Gyte G (1990) The Bristol third stage trial, Teachers' Broadsheet, *New Generation*, Vol 9, No 1, 29.

Harding JE, Elbourne DA, Prendiville PJ (1989) Views of mothers and midwives participating in the Bristol randomised controlled trial of active management of the third stage of labour. *Birth*, Vol 16, No 1, 1-6.

Harris T (2004) Care in the third stage of labour. In: Henderson C, Macdonald S, eds. *Mayes' Midwifery: a textbook for midwives*. 13th edition. London: Bailliere Tindall. Chapter 30, 507-523.

Hastie C (2011) The birthing environment: a sustainable approach. In: Davies L, Daellenbach R, Kensington M, eds. *Sustainability, Midwifery and Birth*. Oxon: Routledge 101-114.

Hemminki E, Marilainen J (1996) Long term effects of caesarean sections: ectopic pregnancies and placental problems. *American Journal of Obstetrics and Gynecology*, Vol 174, 1569-73.

Herschderfer K (1999) Personal Communication to one of the authors. Nadine Edwards.

Hoffman M, Castagnola D, Naqvi F (2006) A randomized trial of active versus expectant management of the third stage of labor [abstract]. *American Journal of Obstetrics and Gynecology*, Vol 195, No 6 Suppl 1: S107.

Hofmery GJ, Gülmezoglu AM, Pileggi C (2010) Vaginal misprostol for cervical ripening and induction of labour. *Cochrane database of systematic reviews*, Issue 10 ART. No.: CD000941.D01:10,1002/14651858.CDD000941.pub2.

Hofmeyr GJ, Gülmezoglu AM (2000) Misoprostol was as efficacious as standard oxytocics for prevention of postpartum hemorrhage. *Evidence-Based Obstetrics and Gynecology*, Vol 2, No 4, 87-88.

Hofmeyr GJ, Neilson JP, Alfirec Z, Crowther CA, Duley L, Gülmezoglu AM, Gyte GML, Hodnett ED (2008) *A Cochrane Pocketbook: Pregnancy and Childbirth*. Chichester: Wiley.

Hofmeyr GJ, Nikodem VC, Jager M, et al (2001) Side-effects of oral misoprostol in the third stage of labour - a randomised placebo-controlled trial. *South African Journal of Obstetrics and Gynaecology*, Vol 7, No 2, 41-42, 44.

Hunt S, Symonds A (1995) *The Social Meaning of Midwifery*. London: Macmillan.

Hutchon DJR (2010) Why do obstetricians and midwives still rush to clamp the cord? *British Medical Journal*, Vol 341 c5447 (Full text available at www.bmj.com/content/341/bmj.c5447.full).

Inch S (1990) Bristol third stage trial commentary. *AIMS Quarterly Journal*, Vol 1, No. 4, 8-10.

Inch S (1989) *Birthrights*. London: Greenprint, Chapter 7, 145-191.

Inch S (1985) Management of the third stage of labour - another cascade of intervention? *Midwifery*, Vol 1, No 2: 114-112.

Inch S (1983) Third stage management *Association of Radical Midwives Newsletter*, No 19, 7-8.

Jackson KW, Allbert JR, Schemmer GK, et al (2001) A randomized controlled trial comparing oxytocin administration before and after placental delivery in the prevention of postpartum hemorrhage. *American Journal of Obstetrics and Gynecology*, Vol 185, No 4, 873-877.

Jerbi M, Hidar S, Elmoueddeb, Chaieb A, Khairi H (2007) Oxytocin in the third stage of labor. *International Journal of Gynecology and Obstetrics*, Vol 96, No 3, 198–9.

Joy SD, Sanchez-Ramos L, Kaunitz AM (August 2003) Misoprostol use during the third stage of labor. *International Journal of Gynecology and Obstetrics*, Vol 82, No 2, 143-152.

Kashanian M, Fekrat M, Masoomi Z, Ansari NS (2010) Comparison of active and expectant management on the duration of the third stage of labour and the amount of blood loss during the third and fourth stage of labour: a randomised controlled trial. *Midwifery*, Vol 26, No 2, 241–5.

Kierse MJNC (1998) What does prevent postpartum haemorrhage? *The Lancet*, 351, March 7, 690-692.

Khan GQ, John IS, Wani S, Doherty T, Sibai BM (1997) Controlled cord traction versus minimal intervention techniques in delivery of the placenta: a randomised controlled trial. *American Journal of Obstetrics and Gynecology*, Vol 177, No 4, 770–4.

Kloosterman G (1975) In: Arms S, *Immaculate Deception*. London: Houghton Mifflin.

Lapido OA (1972) Management of third stage of labour with particular reference to reduction of feto-maternal transfusion. *British Medical Journal*, March 18; 1(5802), 721–72.

Leung SW, Ng PS, Wong WY, et al (2006) A randomised trial of carbetocin versus syntometrine in the management of the third stage of labour. *BJOG: An International Journal of Obstetrics and Gynaecology*, Vol 113, No 12, 1459-1464.

Levy V (1990) The midwife's management of the third stage of labour. In: Alexander J, Levy V, and Roch S, eds. *Midwifery Practice: Intrapartum Care - A Research Based Approach*. London: Macmillan.

Levy V, Moore J (1985) The midwife's management of the third stage of labour. *Nursing Times*, Vol 81, No 5, 47-50.

Lewis G (2007) The Confidential Enquiry into Maternal and Child Health (CEMACH). *Saving Mothers' Lives: reviewing maternal deaths to make motherhood safer 2003-2005. The Seventh Report on Confidential Enquiries into Maternal Deaths in the United Kingdom.* London: CEMACH.

Liabsuetrakul T, Choobun T, Peeyananjarassri K, et al (2007) Prophylactic use of ergot alkaloids in the third stage of labour. *The Cochrane Database of Systematic Reviews*, Issue 2.

Logue M (1990) Management of the third stage of labour: a midwife's view. *Journal of Obstetrics and Gynaecology*, Vol 10, Suppl. 2, 10-12.

Long L (2003) Defining third stage of labour care and discussing optimal practice. *MIDIRS Midwifery Digest*, Vol 13, No 3, 366-370.

Lumbiganon P, Villar J, Piaggio G, et al (2002) Side effects of oral misoprostol during the first 24 hours after administration in the third stage of labour. *BJOG: An International Journal of Obstetrics and Gynaecology*, Vol 109, No 11, 1222-1226.

McDonald S (1999) Physiology and management of the third stage of labour. In: Bennett VR, Brown LK, eds. *Myles Textbook for Midwives* 13th edition. Edinburgh: Churchill Livingstone, 465-488.

McDonald S (2003) Physiology and management of the third stage of labour. In: Fraser DM, Cooper MA, eds. *Myles Textbook for Midwives* 14th edition. Edinburgh: Churchill Livingstone, 507-530.

McDonald S, Abbott JM, Higgins SP (2004) Prophylactic ergometrine-oxytocin versus oxytocin for the third stage of labour (Cochrane Review). (Date of most recent substantive amendment: 25 September 2003) *The Cochrane Database of Systematic Reviews*, Issue 1.

McDonald S, Prendiville WJ, Elbourne DA (1999) Prophylactic syntometrine versus oxytocin for delivery of the placenta. Cochrane Review; last updated: 17 Oct 1996. *In: The Cochrane Library*, Issue 2, Oxford: Update Software.

McDonald SJ, Prendiville W, Blair E (1993) Randomised controlled trial of oxytocin alone versus oxytocin and ergometrine in active management of the third stage of labour. *British Medical Journal* 307, 1167-1171.

Mercer JS (2001) Current best evidence: a review of the literature on umbilical cord clamping. *Journal of Midwifery and Women's Health*, Vol 46, No 6, 402–14.

Mercer JS, Erikson-Owens D (2010) Evidence for neonatal transition and the first hour of life. *In*: Walsh D, Downe S, eds. *Essential midwifery practice: intrapartum care*. Chichester: Wiley, 81-104.

Mercer JS, Nelson CC, Skovgaard RL (2000) Umbilical cord clamping: beliefs and practices of American nurse-midwives. *Journal of Midwifery and Women's Health*, Vol 45, No 1, 58–66.

Mercer JS, Skovgaard R, Erickson-Owens D (2008) Fetal to neonatal transition: first do no harm. *In*: Downe S, ed. *Normal Childbirth: evidence and debate*. 2nd Edition. Edinburgh: Churchill Livingstone, 149–74.

Midwifery Today (1998) *Haemorrhage Special Edition*, No 48.

Muller R, Beck G (1996) Active management of the third stage of labour. *19th Swiss Congress of the Swiss Society of Gynecology and Obstetrics; 1996 June.* Interlaken, Switzerland.

National Childbirth Trust (1993) *The third stage of labour.* (available from the NCT). www.nct.org.uk

Ng PS, Chan ASM, Sin WK, et al (2001) A multicentre randomized controlled trial of oral misoprostol and I.M. syntometrine in the management of the third stage of labour. *Human Reproduction*, Vol 16, No 1, 31-35.

NICE (2007) *Intrapartum care: care of healthy women and their babies during childbirth. NICE clinical guideline 55.* www.nice.org.uk/CG055.

Odent M (2002) *The First Hour Following Birth: Don't Wake the Mother.* www.midwiferytoday.com/articles/firsthour.asp last accessed on 14 March 2011.

Odent M (1999) *The Scientification of Love.* London: Free Association books.

Odent M (1998a) Physiological birth is normal birth, *Midwifery Today Conference 'Keeping Birth Normal'*, London. Sept 10-14.

Odent M (1998b) Don't manage the third stage of labour! *Practising Midwife*, Vol 1, No 9, 31-33.

Orji E, Agwu F, Loto O, et al (2008) A randomized comparative study of prophylactic oxytocin versus ergometrine in the third stage of labor. *International Journal of Gynecology and Obstetrics*, Vol 101, No 2, 129-132.

Parsons SM, Walley RL, Crane JMG, et al (2006) Oral misoprostol versus oxytocin in the management of the third stage of labour. *Journal of Obstetrics and Gynaecology Canada*, Vol 28, No 1, 20-26.

Peyser MR, Kupfermine MJ (1990) Management of severe postpartum haemorrhage by intrauterine irrigation with prostaglandin E2. *American Journal of Obstetrics and Gynaecology*, Vol 1, No. 3.

Porter M, MacIntyre S (1984) What is must be best: a research note on conservative or deferential responses to antenatal care provision. *Social Science and Medicine*, Vol 9, No 11, 1197-1200.

Prendiville WJ, Elbourne DA, McDonald S (1999) Active versus expectant management of the third stage of labour. Cochrane Review; last updated 8 July 1998. In: *The Cochrane Library*, Issue 2. Oxford: Update Software.

Prendiville WJ, Elbourne D, McDonald S. Active versus expectant management in the third stage of labour. *Cochrane Database of Systematic Reviews 2000*, Issue 3. [doi: 10.1002/14651858.CD000007].

Prendiville W, Elbourne D (1989) Care during the third stage of labour. In: Chalmers I, Enkin M, Kierse MJNC, eds. *Effective Care in Pregnancy and Childbirth*. Oxford: Oxford University Press. Vol 2, 1145-1169.

Prendiville WJ, Harding, JE, Elbourne DA (1988) The Bristol third stage trial: active versus physiological management of third stage labour. *British Medical Journal*, Vol 297, 1295-1300.

Prichard K, O'Boyle A, Hogden J (1995) Third stage of labour: outcomes of physiological third stage of labour care in the homebirth setting (November 1991). *New Zealand College of Midwives Journal*, April, 8-10.

Priya JV (1992) *Birth Traditions and Modern Pregnancy Care*. Rockport MA: Element.

Ramirez O, Benito V, Jimenez R, Valido C, Hernandez C, Garcia JA (2001) Third stage of labour: active or expectant management? preliminary results [abstract]. *Journal of Perinatal Medicine*; Suppl 1 (Pt 2), 364.

Razvi K, Chua S, Arulkumaran S, Ratman SS (1996) A comparison between visual estimation of laboratory determination of blood loss during the third stage of labour. *Australian and New Zealand Journal of Obstetrics and Gynaecology*, Vol 36, No 2, 152-154.

RCM (2008) *Third Stage of Labour: Midwifery Practice Guideline*. London: RCM.

Robinson J (1999) *Delivering Your Placenta: The Third Stage*. London: AIMS.

Rogers J (1999) Letter to one of the authors, Nadine Edwards.

Rogers J, Wood J (1999) The Hinchingbrooke third stage trial: what are the implications for practice. *Practising Midwife*, Vol 2, No 2, 35-37.

Rogers J, Wood J, McCandlish R, Ayers S, Truesdale A, Elbourne D (1998) Active versus expectant management of third stage of labour: the Hinchingbrooke randomised controlled trial. *The Lancet*, Vol 351 March 7, 693-699.

Santalahti P, et al (1998) On what grounds to women participate in prenatal screening? *Prenatal Diagnosis*, Vol 18, No 2, 153-165.

Shcmid V (2005) *About physiology in pregnancy and childbirth*. Italy: Firenze.

Singh G, Radhakrishnan G, Guleria K (2009) Comparison of sublingual misoprostol, intravenous oxytocin, and intravenous methylergometrine in active management of the third stage of labor. *International Journal of Gynecology and Obstetrics*, Vol 107, No 2, 130-134.

Sleep J (1989) Physiology and management of the third stage of labour. In: Bennett VR, Brown LK, eds. *Myles Textbook for Midwives* 11th edition. Edinburgh: Churchill Livingstone, 209-222.

Sleep J (1993) Physiology and management of the third stage of labour. In Bennet VR, Brown IK, eds. *Myles Textbook for Midwives* 12th edition. Edinburgh: Churchill Livingstone, Chapter 15, 216-229.

Stevenson J (1989) The Bristol third stage trial. *Association of Radical Midwives Magazine*, No. 4, 11-12.

Stockdale H (1997) Overview of the management of the third stage of labour. *Open Line*, Vol 5, No 3, 9-10, 21-22.

Su LL, Rauff M, Chan YH, et al (2009) Carbetocin versus syntometrine for the third stage of labour following vaginal delivery – a double-blind randomised controlled trial. *BJOG: An International Journal of Obstetrics and Gynaecology*, Vol 116, No 11, 1461-1466.

Sweet BR (1997) Midwifery care in the third stage of labour. In: Sweet BR (ed) *Mayes' Midwifery: A Textbook for Midwives* 12th edition. London: Balliere Tindall. Chapter 31, 403-417.

Thilaganathan B, Cutner A, Latimer J, Beard R (1993) Management of the third stage of labour in women at low risk of postpartum haemorrhage. *European Journal of Obstetrics and Gynaecology and Reproductive Biology*, Vol 48, No 1, 19-22.

Uvnas-Moberg K (2003) *The Oxytocin Factor: Tapping the Hormone of Calm, Love and Healing*. Cambridge, MA: Da Capo Press.

van Dongen PWJ, de Groot ANJA (1995) History of ergot alkaloids from ergotism to ergometrine. *European Journal of Obstetrics and Gynaecology and Reproductive Biology*, Vol 60, No 2, 109-116.

van Teijlingen ER, Hundley V, Rennie AM, Graham W, Fitzmaurice A (2003) Maternity Satisfaction Studies and their limitations: "What is must still be best". *Birth*, Vol 30, No 2, 75-82.

Vasegh FR, Bahiraie A, Mahmoudi M, Salehi L (2005) Comparison of active and physiologic management of third stage of labor. *HAYAT: The Journal of Tehran Faculty of Nursing and Midwifery*, Vol 10, No 23, 102.

Vimala N, Mittal S, Kumar S, et al (2004) Sublingual misoprostol versus methylergometrine for active management of the third stage of labor. *International Journal of Gynecology and Obstetrics*, Vol 87, No1, 1-5.

Walley RL, Wilson JB, Crane JMG and others (2000) A double-blind placebo controlled randomised trial of misoprostol and oxytocin in the management of the third stage of labour. *BJOG: An International Journal of Obstetrics and Gynaecology*, Vol 107, No 9, 1111-1115.

Wangwe P, Kidanto H, Muganyizi P, et al (2009) Active management of third stage of labour: misoprostol or oxytocin? *African Journal of Midwifery and Women's Health*, Vol 3, No 2, 57-60.

Ward A (1983) Syntometrine. *Association of Radical Midwives Newsletter*, No. 18, 21-25.

Watson B (1990) A study of haemoglobin levels in women before and after childbirth. *Midwives Chronicle*, Vol 103, No 1228, 156-158.

Weeks A (2007) Editorial: Umbilical Cord Clamping After Birth. *British Medical Journal*, Vol 335, 312.

Welsh G (1997) Wisdom of the midwives: postpartum bleeding. *Midwifery Today*, No 42, 13.

Wesson N (1990) *Homebirth*. London: Macdonald Optima.

Wesson N (2006) *Home Birth: A Practical Guide*. London: Pinter and Martin.

Wickham S (1999) Further thoughts on the third stage. *Practising Midwife*, Vol 8, No 11, 37.

Wickham S (2001) *Anti-D in Midwifery: Panacea or Paradox*. Edinburgh: Books for Midwives.

Wickham S (2005) The birth of water embolism. *Practising Midwife*, Vol 8, No 11, 37.

Wickham S (2010) Research Unwrapped. *Practising Midwife*, Vol 3, No 2, 31-32.

Wickham S, Robinson D (2010) Nil nocere: doing no harm as an important guiding principle within maternity care. *MIDIRS Midwifery Digest*, Vol 20, No 4, 415-420.

Wood J, Rogers J (1997) The third stage of labour. *In*: Alexander J, Levy V, Roth C eds. *Midwifery Practice: Core Topics 2*. London: Macmillan Press Ltd, 113-126.

Wolford MC (1997) First do no harm. *Midwifery Today*, 15-17.

World Health Organisation (1996) *Care in normal birth: a practical guide, Report of a Technical Working Group*. WHO/FRH/MSM/96.24, Geneva.

Yoa AC, Lind J (1974) Placental transfusion. *American Journal of 7Diseases in Children*, Vol 127, 128-141.

Zachariah ES, Naidu M, Seshadri L (2006) Oral misoprostol in the third stage of labor. *International Journal of Gynecology and Obstetrics*, Vol 92, No 1, 23-26.

Zaki M, et al (1998) Risk factors and morbidity in patients with placenta previa accreta compared to placenta previa non-accreta. *Acta Obstetrica Gynecologica Scandinavia*, Vol 77, 391-94.

Zenack M (1998) *Lotus Birth*. Birthkit, 18: 6.

AIMS - Association for Improvements in Maternity Services

Was the information in this book helpful to you?

Please let us know your views of this book. Particularly, if you think there is information that could be included, or amended. Send your views to:
Chair@aims.org.uk

Other Publications

Other publications published by AIMS, many of which can be ordered via PayPal on the AIMS web site: www.aims.org.uk

- Am I Allowed?
- Birth After Caesarean
- Birthing Your Baby
- Breech Birth
- Home Birth
- Induction
- Making a Complaint
- Ultrasound Unsound?
- Vitamin K
- Water Birth
- What's Right for Me
- AIMS Quarterly Journals

About AIMS

The Association for Improvements in the Maternity Services (AIMS) has been in the forefront of the childbirth movement for the last fifty years. Our day to day work includes providing independent support and information about maternity choices and raising awareness of current research on childbirth and related issues. AIMS actively supports parents and healthcare professionals who recognise that, for the majority of women, birth is a normal rather than a medical event.

There are no paid staff in AIMS, every member gives her/his time voluntarily, if this information has helped you, please help us to continue our work by joining AIMS or make a donation to help us continue to help others. You can join or donate via our web site www.aims.org.uk

Association for Improvements in the Maternity Services (AIMS), 5 Ann's Court, Grove Road, Surbiton, Surrey, KT6 4BE.
Tel: 0202 8390 9534. helpline@aims.org.uk